Learning

Exact Blueprint on How to Learn Faster and Remember Anything Memory, Study Skills & How to Learn

Learning

© Copyright 2015 - All rights reserved.

In no way is it legal to reproduce, duplicate, or transmit any part of this document in either electronic means or in printed format. Recording of this publication is strictly prohibited and any storage of this document is not allowed unless with written permission from the publisher. All rights reserved.

The information provided herein is stated to be truthful and consistent, in that any liability, in terms of inattention or otherwise, by any usage or abuse of any policies, processes, or directions contained within is the solitary and utter responsibility of the recipient reader. Under no circumstances will any legal responsibility or blame be held against the publisher for any reparation, damages, or monetary loss due to the information herein, either directly or indirectly.

Respective authors own all copyrights not held by the publisher.

Legal Notice:

This book is copyright protected. This is only for personal use. You cannot amend, distribute, sell, use, quote or paraphrase any part or the content within this book without the consent of the author or copyright owner. Legal action will be pursued if this is breached.

Disclaimer Notice:

Please note the information contained within this document is for educational and entertainment purposes only. Every attempt has been made to provide accurate, up to date and reliable complete information. No warranties of any kind are expressed or implied. Readers acknowledge that the author is not engaging in the rendering of legal, financial, medical or professional advice.

Learning

By reading this document, the reader agrees that under no circumstances are we responsible for any losses, direct or indirect, which are incurred as a result of the use of information contained within this document, including, but not limited to, —errors, omissions, or inaccuracies.

Table of Contents

Bonus	ix
Introduction	x
Chapter 1: Memory	1
Primary Memory	2
Secondary Memory	3
Chapter 2: Memory Tool-Kit	6
Stage I	6
Stage II	8
Watch What You put in Your Mouth	8
Meditation is the Key	10
How does Meditation help?	11
How do I meditate?	11
Getting out of meditation	19
Chapter 3: Physical Fitness And Memory	20
Stage III	21
Chapter 4: Memory Enhancement For Students	23
Attention Span Enhancement	23
Staying Alert	24
Meals	25
Read To Understand, Not Mug Up	27
Familiarity Breeds Memory	28
Use Literary Devices	29
Buzzwords	29
Acronyms	30
Acrostics	30
Method of Loci	31

Learning

Parts	32
Rhymes and Rhythms	32
Association	33
Flash cards	33
Chapter 5: Imagination And Memory	35
Chapter 6: Ask And You Shall Learn	40
Chapter 7: Self-Explanation	44
Chapter 8: Summarization	46
Chapter 9: Study Cycling	50
Chapter 10: Keyword Mnemonic	52
Chunking	52
Graphics	53
Learning Passwords	53
Chapter 11: Idea Mapping	54
Cloud-Circle-Flowchart Idea Map	55
Tree Branch Idea Map	56
Idea Mapping Benefits	57
Chapter 12: How Idea Mapping Can Be Useful in Learning	59
Memorization	59
Boosting Creativity	61
Note taking	61
Revising	62
Brainstorming	64
Summarizing content	66
Presentations & reports	67
To-do lists	68

Learning

Problem Solving And Decision Making	70
Student Assessment and group projects	72
Managing information	72
Chapter 13: Reading For Learning	**75**
Survey	75
Question	77
Read	78
Review	79
Raising The Bar	80
Chapter 14: Speed Reading	**81**
Poor Reading Habit #1: Sub-Vocalization	82
Poor Reading Habit #2: Word Reading	83
Poor Reading Habit #3: Eye Motion	84
Poor Reading Habit #4: Regressing	84
Poor Reading Habit #5: Being Distracted	85
How Fast (Or Slow) Do We Read?	86
Goal Setting	87
Ready, Get Set, Speed!	88
Keep Your (Mental) Mouth Shut	89
Cover Operations	89
Efficient Eye Movements	90
Speed Brain Training	91
Skim Reading	92
Visual Representations	93
Chapter 15: Note Taking	**95**
Chapter 16: Interleaved Practice	**97**
Is It Effective?	98

Learning

How Does It Work?	98
Practical Tips For Using Interleaved Practice	100
Chapter 17: Self-Assessment	102
Chapter 18: Self-Monitoring	105
Chapter 19: Asking Questions	107
Chapter 20: Listen Actively	110
Chapter 21: Teach It To Learn It	116
Chapter 22: Other High Efficiency Study Methods	118
Practice Testing	118
Distributed Practice	119
Elaborative Interrogation	120
Highlighting	121
Rereading	121
Think-Pair-Share	122
Question Stacking	123
The Exit Ticket	123
Active Learning	124
Just-in-time Teaching	124
Listening Teams	125
Structured Sharing	126
Chapter 23: Lifestyle	130
Stress	130
Sleep	139
Socials	140

Learning

Chapter 24: How to Eat To Boost Your Memory and Learning	143
Conclusion	158
Bonus	159

Learning

Bonus

Thanks for making it this far in your education. If you want the real multiplier effect and to take your skills and effectiveness to the next level, I recommend the easy-to-follow quick tips below.

[CLICK HERE: Top 10 Productivity Tips & Hacks GUARANTEED to Unlock Massive Amounts of Time, Crush Decision Fatigue, and Skyrocket Your Efficiency and Effectiveness](https://funnelb.leadpages.co/smarter-not-harder-business/)

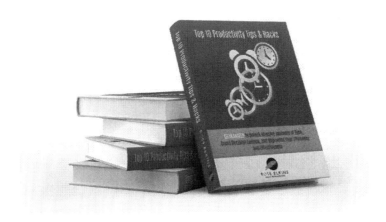

Link: https://funnelb.leadpages.co/smarter-not-harder-business/

Learning

Introduction

Have you found yourself forgetting things? Are you someone who travels all the way to the kitchen, opens the fridge only to fidget at what you were there for in the first place? If yes, then you have purchased the right book!

I want to congratulate you for choosing the key to maintaining a perfect memory throughout your life. We are going to deal with the various ways in which you can not only keep your static memory intact, but also extend the reach of your memorizing powers beyond levels you cannot even fathom.

Forgetting things is as common as catching a cold. You tend to forget many things in a day. It could be something as simple as paying the newspaper guy his monthly fees or something as disastrous as attending an urgent office meeting. Not everyone is perfect when it comes to keeping track of things that they are supposed to remember and follow up with an action through the day.

Forgetting is as human as being selfish. Yet, we need to get rid of this habit in order to move further in life in the smoothest way possible. Forgetting might sound like such a common mistake to do but in reality, it leads us to drastic results when the instances of you forgetting important matters are piled up.

This book is aimed at giving you the best methods to get rid of this habit and to improve your memory to an extent from where it is impossible to simply forget something. You will be equipped with various ways, which will help your life take a U turn from monotonous and nonchalant

Learning

to exciting and alert. You do not have to be a cat in order to keep your tail up anything that comes your way.

You will be walked through time-tested techniques on how to enhance your memory, especially with regards to academics and generally the daily life. You no longer have to worry about the mess you end up creating due to your annoying habit of forgetting things that matter. In simple words, after having read this book, your life will be headed towards a major change.

Without further ado, let us begin our journey!

Learning

Chapter 1: Memory

Welcome to the first chapter of this book. Just as most first chapters do, this one will be dedicated towards making you familiar with the concept and variations of the concept of memory. This chapter will lay the foundation of everything that you are going to encounter in the next few chapters.

Let us start with what memory really is. We use the word 'memory' in our daily lives, just like we use the word 'please', 'excuse', and 'pollution'. It is as common a word as any other. Have you ever paused for awhile and thought about what it really is? Let us get you familiar with the real dynamics of memory functioning.

In purely psychological terms, memory is a place. It is a place where information, of any kind, is stored, processed and retrieved whenever required. Imagine a large palace adorned with chandeliers and containing a lot of rooms, smaller than the bigger hall that stands in the middle.

Psychologists refer to this place as the human Memory Palace. A Memory Palace is nothing but a hypothetical place, which has been constructed to give you an idea of how memory functions. The small rooms that the palace contains are mere divisions of your memory according to classifications unconsciously made by you. One room could be about your office meeting timings, submission of important documents and salary details. This room is specifically meant for one-purpose only - office related memories.

Another room could be filled with memories associated with your romantic interest. Sarah and her face pictures, the gown that you gifted her and the romantic dinner dates you have been on together- this room will be overflowing with memories related to your love life. There will be another room that will be filled with embarrassing stories from your past.

Remember that one time in high school when you bent down to pick your pen and your pants ripped? Or the date you went to, with pimples adorning your face like flies. This room is seldom opened and stays usually locked. There could be another room filled with your life's fantasies. We all have fantasies we do not admit having. You could have a particular fetish when it comes to sex and you are too scared to admit it to your partner. You store such fetishes in a single room inside your memory palace. Hence, a memory palace is a collection of everything that you have experienced and you wish to achieve.

Now that you have been made familiar with a general understanding of how your memory functions, let us move ahead and have a good grasp about the real and most accurate idea of memory- the biological understanding of it.

Your memory can be classified into two divisions- Primary and Secondary.

Primary Memory

Primary memory is nothing but a collection of everything and anything that has a short life span. Imagine driving through the traffic to your office and reading a billboard on the way. It features Pamela Anderson in her famous beachwear. You will look at it for a minute, read the accompanying product that she is trying to sell, hear the honks from behind and move ahead towards the direction of your workplace. By the time you are back home in the evening, having a meal, you would not remember what exact product Pam was trying to sell, or what colored beach wear did she wear while doing it. This is your short-term memory.

A person's short-term memory contains information related to things that have just happened. Such things are not important to the person's life, not now at least. Short-term memory helps you move through the day though. The bits of information it provides you with ultimately forms links to join together and lead to the forging of the large chain that pulls you through your day. Imagine if you started forgetting the tiniest of details about what you just did. Remember the example given at the start of this book about the fridge? That is one of the best instances of the disadvantages of short-term memory loss.

Secondary Memory

Long-term memory on the other hand, is obviously wider than short-term memory. Look at how I used the word wider and not better. We will come to this later. Long-term memory is the collection of all those memories that you have stored in order to retrieve later in life. Such memories are not easily washed away by stress or daily life shenanigans. There are certain things in life that you cannot just simply forget about. These things could range from the first time you had sex to your social security number.

Studies have shown that the long-term memory of a person is naturally stronger than his short-term memory. The contents of your long-term memory are close and dear to you. The contents could also be simply important without having any sort of emotional worth to you or your life. The more the contents of a long-term memory of a person, the healthier his memory in general is. In fact, one of the surest ways to gauge how strong someone's memory is to have a look at how big one's long term memory department is.

There is another form of memory that you need to understand before advancing further in this book. Scientifically called Sensory memory, this type of memory is even shorter than your short-term memory. It is the shortest possible form of memory. You must be familiar with the five basic humans senses. Smell, sight, taste, touch and listening! The basic five human sensations contribute to ninety percent of whatever experiences you go through in your life. Everything else is mostly psychological in nature. Sensory memory stores the immediate information that you gather by the employment of these five senses. Imagine walking down the street to buy groceries. Due to the locality being a suburb, there would be drug peddler trying to sell you cheap drugs. One such rag picker comes up to you and tries to sell something wrapped in white polythene. Although you are not someone who is into such illegal indulgences, you have a look at the teenager rag picker and scrounge your nose to show disappointment and disinterest in his offer. You walk off your way after having made a signal that you do not want the drugs. However, after reaching the grocery, you still retain the details about the person's appearance, with regards to his clothes, appeal and the contents of his hands.

This is your sensory memory helping you recall whatever you experienced only minutes ago. Sensory memory can work in seconds as well. It helps you recall the minutest possible things in your day-to-day lives.

So it all comes down to how well you are able to apply the knowledge you acquired in the chapter to efficient use in your lives. No amount of knowledge is useful unless it is successfully applied to give you gains in life. Hence it is important that the useful inputs you amassed in this

Learning

chapter be converted into useful output. The next chapters will deal with the various ways in which you can sharpen your different classes of memory. For now though, I hope you have retained whatever you have read till now. Keep whatever you read in mind while treading further. Let us march ahead and learn how best to enhance our memory and lead ourselves to a smarter life.

Chapter 2: Memory Tool-Kit

Welcome to the second chapter of this book. Here we shall explore all the possible ways to not just enhance your memory and take it to extreme levels of excellence but also maintain it in its peak form without compromising on anything important in your lives. Your memory, as has been described in the last chapter, is more of a place than an organ. How do you make sure that a place is in its prime form? You dust it and then start renovating it. This chapter will teach you exactly that. Let us begin our journey towards a better life.

Memory Enhancement is a process that has been split into three stages. These three stages must be gone though in the exact order they have been enlisted otherwise the very point will be defeated in the run. Let us explore the first stage.

Stage I

Stage I involves everything that can help your memory prepare itself to receive the memory training you are going to impart. Imagine a kid going to school the first time ever. Do you directly admit him to the said school and expect him to start rotting up mathematics table? No. You prepare him for the experience. You make sure that he is ready to receive education before he is enrolled into an educational institution. Maybe admitting him to a nursery or a kindergarten would help. You slowly ease him into the experience of academics.

Stage I majorly consists of baby steps that are taken in order to ready your brain for the eventual procedure. When you move into a new house, you do not start arranging your things right after moving in. You dust off

Learning

the place, make sure the shelves are clean and ensure hygiene before letting your kids play around or things moved into the house. Your memory is no different. Let us learn how.

Your memory could be prevented from being on top due to a variety of reasons. There could be many factors contributing to your memory being slowed and tied down. Stage I is where you are to take steps necessary to make sure that such hindrances are removed from your path.

You could start off with removing emotional attachment from things in general. Being sentimentally inclined towards a thing or a person blind your memory. When you develop partial feelings towards an entity, you naturally get more inclined towards it than other things in your life. As a result, you end up devoting a major part of your mental energy towards this entity rather than equally distributing it amongst everything. This leads to an imbalance and hence imperfections in your memory. For example, let's assume that James' favorite subject is mathematics. He can be seen around his college campus, solving sums and making derivations. However, due to his overt enthusiasm for the subject, he is unable to devote as much energy towards history. As a predictable result, his history marks suffer. He is not able to recall important historical dates as easily as he'd mathematical formulas. This happened because he was more inclined towards one subject than the rest; so much so that after a point he no longer felt the passion for the rest of the subjects thereby losing his interest in them.

Excessive leaning towards anything is a bad thing and must be gotten rid of. You should be emotional, yes, but being partially emotional you are pushing yourself towards doom. Memory is directly related to emotions. The more emotionally attached you are to an entity; the more imbalanced your memory is going to be. Of course some things are supposed to be more important than the others, but an abundance of attention and energy when dedicated to just one leads to negligence and substantial cutting off of the rest.

Stage I is very important as it prepares your mind to let go of things you would not have previously. Letting go is a major part of just not memory enhancement but moving ahead in life as well. So long as you hold on to your past, you are not going to be able to even take the first step towards improving your memory.

Stage II

The most important of the three steps, Stage II is about applying direct methods to improve your memory. This step will span over a longer area than the rest two because of how vital and necessary it is. The real crux of this book is hidden in this step, so I'd urge you to pay your utmost attention here.

Watch What You put in Your Mouth

Food is life! A simple activity of our daily routine, eating is usually not considered a very important phenomenon in our lives. However, if you want to make sure that your memory is improving, you must pay close attention to what is there on your plate. Your food is the first key to your memory enhancement. Here is a list of some food items that are a must if you are looking forward to an excellent memory:

Tomatoes are a sure shot way to memory improvement. Tomatoes contain sufficient carbohydrates, vitamin A and C, potassium and anti-oxidants. Not only are they rich in the aforementioned elements, they also help your skin glow, which in turn could be a confidence boost to your personality, thereby helping you with remembering things in general.

Coffee is another source of valuable contents that help your memory. Caffeine has been proved to have helped students' not just stay up long hours at nights, but also develop their short-term memory. Researchers are unclear as to the exact reason behind caffeine helping young guns prepare for exams. It could be because of how it helps you stay up or that the caffeine has the necessary compounds to really enhance your short-term memory, or a mixture of both. Either way, coffee is a must for long nights.

Fish is rich in omega three fatty acids, which are excellent for optimum brain and memory functioning. Eating fish at least once a week is good enough to provide your brain the aforementioned omega three fatty acids. The oil present in the fish is also very good for short-term memory retention.

Munching on **walnuts** is also a helpful tip to improve your memory. Walnuts and other related nuts like peanuts and the like contain omega three fatty acids in abundant amounts. Moreover, they are also rich in elegiac acid, which is a sure shot protective element when it comes to free radical damage to the brain.

You must have heard about the powers of **rosemary oil**. You would be surprised to know the way in which rosemary oil helps you when it comes to memory. You could use rosemary oil to help your memory by burning it and leaving it to spread its essence in your house. It is said that the essence of rosemary oil when burnt somehow helps you memorize things quicker. You can also use the oil in cooking and other food items. Along with **olive oil** rosemary oil adds to the aftertaste of many food items.

Turkey, an important food during thanksgiving, is also a good memory booster. When properly roasted, turkey lets out L-Tyrosine, an element that helps you improve mental alertness. It does not let you ignore that matter to you and your overall alertness is increased twice the amount. L-Tyrosine can also be found in yogurt, cheese and chicken.

Choline, a precursor of acetylcholine, can be found in eggs. Eggs besides being really tasty food choices can also help you on your way to memory improvement. Acetylcholine is a neuro-stimulator that helps pass on messages from one nerve ending to another. When you have abundant amounts of acetylcholine in your system, you tend to be more alert when you are surrounded by distractions.

Note: We will discuss more of this in the last chapter to help you understand how what you eat affects your memory.

Meditation is the Key

Few people recognize the potential of a good meditation session. Meditation can be best described as the shutting down of all the senses for a while before letting your mind focus on one point, irrespective how the number of distractions wandering around you. Meditation is an ancient art of clearing out your thoughts and paying attention to only that which is importune to you. Saints and sages from the past have always recommended it and so are yoga gurus these days. The importance of meditation cannot be put into words. It improves not just your memory but also your health. Doctors have begun acknowledging the value of a good meditation over medication. Medical practitioners around the world have come to recognize meditation as a full proof medical practice to get rid of things that couldn't have been cured by general branches of allopathic medicine.

How does Meditation help?

Meditation is nothing but focusing your entire attention pool to one point and not letting distractions sway your focus. With regards to how it helps your memory, it has been established that when you focus all your energy to a single point, you learn self-control and focus. Self-focus and self-control are two such things that can anyway sharpen your memory like a whetstone sharpens a sword. When you are equipped in handling your energy according to where you want it to focus, you naturally learn how to control it. Gaining control over your attention radar is a major achievement. Once you have gained this said control, you have improved your memory by half of what it used to be. Meditation is therefore, a proven technique to help you improve your memory.

How do I meditate?

You do not have to wander around to some countryside, find a big tree and sit under it trying to focus your energies. You really do not need any special place for meditation. Although meditation can be performed really anywhere, for beginners, it is advised that they follow some tips in order to successfully meditate. Let me share some of these tips with you:

Choose a quiet place for meditation. This place could be anywhere, like for example your personal study room, your office cabin or even a park. Just make sure that the room or the place you have chosen is free for the next one hour.

Learning

Make sure that you are not hindering in anyone's activity while you are occupying the space you have selected for meditating.

Assume a cross-legged position and sit down on the floor. Floor is preferred over any other place to sit while meditating because a cross-legged position on the floor has been proved to be the best position to meditate. This is said to elevate all your senses to their maximum level.

Before assuming the mentioned position, mark a point on the opposite wall. This point will be the point of your focus. It is a very important step for beginners since they will need a reference point to focus their energies on. As soon as you are done performing this step with the help of a pencil or a dark marker, get back to your sitting position.

Start your meditation by looking at the marked spot with a clear vision. Start off easy. Do not focus too much of your attention on the spot as it may lead to severe headache after some hours.

Make sure you remove any sort of distraction from the place you are meditating in. When you do that, you ensure that no one or nothing proves a disturbance to you while you are trying to focus.

When you have looked at the mark for long enough, try looking at it with more focus now. Do not, however, squint your eyes as this may lead to acute issues of headache later. Focus with a normal gaze and try to muster all your vision to that particular spot only.

Important note:

Switch off your mobile phone before starting the session. Bolt the doors and the windows so that even a car honk or a buzzing fly would not be able to take your mind off the spot. The purpose of isolating you while you are focusing is to make sure you become an expert at separating things eventually. Deliberate isolation is helpful only at the start, hence the bolting of the doors and the windows. But after you have gained some mastery over focusing yourself on the said spot, try to keep the doors and the windows open, thereby challenging your focus. If you have reached a stage where even the loudest ring of your mobile is not able to distract you from your spot, know that you are progressing.

When you perform this, you enhance the energies in your body. Chakras that are supposed to be your pressure points are in their peaks and you experience liberation of a different kind altogether. You not only are at the peak of your senses but also your powers of imagination.

After you have focused on the spot, for about an hour, you can gradually start focusing on different things in your environment. For example, try looking at how pretty the vase kept in the corner of the room is, or try smiling at the photo of your kid hung up on the wall, just above the spot you were just so focused on. Do not suddenly snap out of your meditation as it could lead to issues. Make the way out gradual and simple.

Do you want to make your meditation session more creative, fun, and relaxing? Why not try bath meditation, aromatherapy, and other intriguing techniques? Let's see how you can do that:

- **Bath Meditation**

You can try this technique to obtain the benefits from a relaxing and soothing hot bath that allows tiredness and stress to be released from your muscles. To make such a bath meditation set-up, refer to this guideline:

-Make time for meditation, such as 15 minutes of uninterrupted practice. Buy a few aromatherapy-bathing products such as peppermint or lavender scented soap to make stress relief more effective.

-Get into the bath water and relax. Allow your breathing to be deeper and slower, allow your belly to rise and fall naturally with the breathing patterns.

-Pay your attention to the sensations that come from your body, such as the warmth of the water on your skin or the pressure the tub exerts on your back. Release your thought, keep the mind calm as you try to focus as much as possible to the present moment.

-Continue with the bath meditation, for a few minutes, until you feel soothed and well relaxed. Ensure that thoughts of the past or internal dialogue do not affect your concentration.

- **Chocolate Meditation**

Everyone likes chocolate and why not get creative about it? This is a very pleasurable form of meditation that is very easy to commit to especially because it has chocolate as the reward! Dark chocolate is nutritious and doesn't cause those undesired feelings associated with other sugary snacks. Here are the steps you can follow to meditate with chocolate:

✓ Get a bite-sized piece of dark chocolate with a large content of cocoa or semi-sweet chips or chocolate kiss.

✓ Relax your body and take slow and deep breaths, while closing your eyes.

✓ Take a small chocolate bite and then allow it to sit on your tongue as it melts into the mouth.

Concentrate on the sensations coming from chocolate flavors, as you continue with deep breathing.

- ✓ Swallow slowly focusing on how the chocolate goes down, and how the mouth later feels empty.

- ✓ Take another bite, and focus on how the arm feels when bringing the chocolate to your mouth, the feelings between your fingers and how it gets into your mouth. Also focus on the feelings it's causing at the present moment.

- ✓ As in other meditation practices, control those interrupting thoughts coming into your mind throughout your chocolate meditation, and then refocus on the sensations or flavors in the present moment.

- ✓ Savor the feeling, ensuring to revisit this feeling in your entire day so that you feel more relaxed and happy. You may either continue with the meditation without the chocolate or resume your daily tasks afterwards.

- **Meditate With Aromatherapy**

Aromatherapy is a way of utilizing the natural oils extracted from plants to improve the physical and psychological well-being. As a form of therapy, you stand to benefit from a relaxed mind, body, and soul. Even if you are new to meditation, you can easily create an easy aromatherapy session. Follow this guideline:

- ✓ Adopt a relaxed posture and then light a stick of incense such as lavender stick incense, following the package directions

Learning

- ✓ Wait for trails of smoke to curl and waft upwards and then watch the smoke. Just allow your mind to be immersed in the various patterns or paths that the smoke trails take.

- ✓ Do not allow other thoughts to come into your mind, by trying to bring your attention to the trails coming from the incense. Wait for a moment, and appreciate the elegant and simple display.

- ✓ You can inhale the refreshing aroma as much as possible, based on your ability to focus. To start with, you can try 5-10 minutes a number of times per week, and later try daily for a longer duration of 30 minutes.

- ✓ Try lavender, peppermint, and sage scents but be careful not to have the smoke trails too close to your eyes or nose. If you have respiratory problem with burning incense, you may do other meditation practices instead.

- **Breathing meditation**

Deep breathing is another relaxing technique that focuses on full cleansing breaths. The practice is easy to learn and can be done at any place, and can offer a fast way to control your stress levels. Deep breathing is the cornerstone in most relaxation techniques such as music or aromatherapy. To practice breathing meditation, you'll only require a place to stretch out plus a few minutes.

The key to breathing deeply is doing it from the abdomen in order to get as much fresh air as possible from the lungs. Once you take deep breaths from your abdomen,

Learning

you'll inhale more oxygen as opposed from shallow breaths from the upper chest. And the more oxygen that gets into your system, the less tense, anxious and out of breath you feel.

- ✓ Sit comfortably, preferably with your back straight. Place one of your hands on the chest and the other on the stomach.

- ✓ Start breathing through the nose, where the hand placed on the stomach should rise with the diaphragm. However, the other hand on the chest should only move slightly.

- ✓ Then exhale through the mouth, and ensure that you push maximum amount of air as you contract the abdominal muscles. As you exhale, the hand placed on your stomach should move in.

- ✓ Continue with the breathing exercise through the nose, and exhale through the mouth. When you exhale, do it in such a way that the lower abdomen raises and falls. You can count 1-5 as you exhale.

In case you find it harder to breathe from the abdomen from a standing position, you can lie comfortably on the floor. Try placing a book on your stomach and watch it rise and fall as you breathe.

- **Visualization meditation**

This meditation technique works in two ways. First, it brings you closer to the positive end-state that you desire and helps you rid yourself out of the problems or negativity that results into stress or anxiety. Practice the technique regularly for better results through these simple steps:

Learning

- ✓ Sit in a comfortable meditation posture, and then close your eyes. Take a few deep breaths from your diaphragm and ensure that you relax your stomach.

- ✓ Now imagine being at a scenery with radiant white light. Take your time to experience the light that fills you with the serenity and bliss.

- ✓ Inhale this imaginary brilliant light with each breath that you take, and allow the light to be absorbed in your entire body. This light should wash your entire organs, reach every cell, and then suffuse every atom of your body. At the end of the practice, you should be fully absorbed in it.

- ✓ To deal with an emotion or other negative thoughts, visualize yourself exhaling the negativity out, in a form of thick black smoke. Try to achieve your desired state of mind and then focus on the way you would feel after achieving it. As you visualize the good feeling, inhale that image with every breath you take.

For better results, make the image as detailed or real as possible, by incorporating real colors, smell, sounds, and feelings.

Memory is directly linked to how well you focus. Normally, your attention span is weak and you do not really remember everything that you see. Either that, or you try to remember everything and retain nothing. Meditating heightens your senses to unimaginable levels and makes you the master of your attention. You will realize that once you have gained control over what you want to see what you don't, things start becoming simpler for you. What used to bother you before is no longer such an issue anymore. You start seeing yourself in a new light since the senses that you have mastered are now your servants and

Learning

hence, so is your memory, which has grown sharper, better and stronger.

Getting out of meditation

At the end of a meditation session, you need to give yourself enough time. The way you "get out" matters a lot just like the actual meditation. The main point of meditation is to carry the relaxed focus into action. To properly exit the meditation mood without affecting the relaxed state of mind, follow these steps:

1. Be aware that you indeed want to end your meditation soon, i.e. the body should appreciate that within a few seconds, you would get up. From here, your body should be relaxed to shift gears from the healing mood back to the neutral gear.

2. Don't do anything. The state of mind allows you to let thoughts come and go, and sensations follow the same path; without you intending anything. You can take around 1-3 minutes, which is indeed a long time worth a whole world of experience. To help you take a longer time, you might need a timer or alarm clock.

3. As you approach the moment to get out of meditation, make small movements such as a sigh. Wait for a moment then repeat the same little movement. This should help you feel your metabolism start to speed up.

4. You can now open your eyes a little, then close them briefly and realize your inner feelings. If necessary, sigh again and open the eyes. Try to look downwards and in front of yourself for a moment, as your eyelids may not have to open all the way.

5. Finally open the eyes and then sit there for 30 seconds, as you savor your mood sensations.

Learning

Chapter 3: Physical Fitness And Memory

It is a fact that your body is directly related to your mental health. Your memory is not going to enhance itself. You are going to have to do it, and one of the proven techniques is to make sure that your body is in prime form. I am not talking about hitting the gym and aiming for six packs in three months. I am talking about staying fit, though flabby and without muscle. Being physically fit has been mistaken for turning into Ryan gosling for too long now. The myth needs to be shattered, as you can be physically fit without looking so.

When you are physically healthy, your mind picks up the signal and tries to improve itself. It is a biological phenomenon that your mind's health is directly related to your body. Of course, it is not necessary that you develop a six-packs, but it would not hurt to have one either. For the same, you must hit the local gym and exercise yourself to death.

You can choose to stay physically fit by improving your plate. Do not go for oily and fatty food, as all you get from such food items is fat and acids, which are harmful for your memory. Recurring disease are also an important contributor towards memory degradation. You can improve memory in two ways - by enhancing it from zero, or by removing factors that take it to below zero.

Sometimes, your memory is below zero by default, even before you realize that your memory is bad. Hence, it is important you start alienating those factors that are taking your memory down. Start with the cleansing process by first bringing it to zero and then dream of taking it further

Learning

from there. For the same, get rid of your unhealthy food choices.

Like it is said above, no oily food items should form a part of your diet. Go for boiled and steamed food over fried or roasted food. Boiling and steaming are such cooking processes that waste the minimum of essential natural nutrients of the food subjected to boiling or steaming. After a vegetable is boiled, it retains almost all its original nutrients that are beneficial to you. However, when fried or roasted, or subjected to any process that involves the employment of heat, the essential elements of a natural food product are destroyed. Remember, fire destroys while ice preserves.

Stage III

Stage three of the memory enhancement process largely consists of steps taken to make sure whatever you have learned stays with you. It is a step that is based on the principles of retention. In order to be sure that the ways you followed to improve your memory are not un-followed after a few weeks of religious devotion, here are enlisted certain tips to be followed:

- You have to have a certain amount of self-belief so as to survive the process of memory enhancement. Without you believing in yourself regarding the process of memory retention, you cannot simply hope to enhance your memory.

- Besides self-belief, a substantial level of self-confidence also goes into your memory improvement. Unless you are confident about retaining things that matter to you in general, memory improvement remains a dream that is yet to be fulfilled.

- Stage third of memory enhancement helps you make the entire procedure more solid in terms of retention. When you seal the deal, you make sure that whatever you learned from the procedure stays with you for longer than a predictable amount of time.

The three prescribed stages of memory enhancement are numbered for a reason. You must perform in whole the first stage before advancing into the second and so on. Make sure your mind is prepared to take the efforts to be put in for improvement of your memory. Do not rush into the entire process without first readying yourself for it.

Although there are no noticeable adverse reactions, the chances of receiving efficient outputs get decreased to substantial levels. The process that has been given above is a wholesome one. You cannot expect results out of it by simply going through them as if you are reading the morning newspaper. You need to be dedicated towards improving your memory. The steps so written are only a skeleton work and are in no way exhaustive. You could tweak them according to your own circumstances and convenience.

However, if you thought religiously performing the process would be enough, you are in for a rude awakening. There is no sure shot way to improving your memory overnight. You need to understand that these are only suggestions gathered from the experiences of those who have suffered memory issues in the past, survived them and made it out to clinch success in the end. This chapter was not an encyclopedia of memory tips, but rather the success story of those who have suffered the same hurdles as you. If they could beat the odds, I don't see a reason for you not to.

Learning

Chapter 4: Memory Enhancement For Students

Welcome to the fourth chapter of the book. This section will deal with those classes of our readers who are in immediate need of a memory boost - students. Though the previous chapters are equally helpful for those pursuing any course in education, this chapter is more specific in nature when it comes to proving useful for students.

Students are the kind of crowd you would get everywhere. It does not matter which country you are from or what sort of standard of living you are accustomed to; if you are a student, you are surely going to benefit from this chapter.

Students, by the very nature of what they are supposed to do, are certainly in need of anything that has been prescribed here. It is their constant struggle to keep themselves updated with facts, figures, theories and ideas. Academics are an important phase of anyone's life and must not be ignored and left to average performance. If you want to excel in academics, the first requirement that you must cater to is a good and sharp memory.

It is a general complaint of any average student that they are not able memorizes things right on time. Even if they do, they are not able to retain it beyond a particular time, and this time usually stops at the first week after the first reading. Below are some useful tricks to keep your memory up and running even if the number of times you have read your material is few.

Attention Span Enhancement

Attention span can be best described as the amount and radius of focus you dedicate towards particular thing. Your attention span is usually measured in seconds and does not exceed three seconds on an average. The amount of time you spend on observing something can also be summarized as your attention span. The more your attention span, the more the time you spend memorizing something. The very basis of memory improvement is that you spend enough time trying to understand a subject.

If you want to improve your memory, you need to improve your attention span. Do not simply turn your head after looking at something that is supposed to be important. Spend enough time observing the thing's behavior, peculiarities, exceptional qualities and anomalies. When you consume something in whole, you are bound to retain a major portion of it, as opposed to when you consume the same thing in portions and bits thereby retaining only a smaller amount of the same.

Staying Alert

Believe it or not, if you have a bad memory, most probably you are also suffering from a dull mind. Alertness is of prime importance when it comes to memory improvement. When your mind is dull and is shut down by something grave, you tend to stay less alert than usual. A lack of alertness can be caused by a range of factors that need to be eliminated, before you could move further down the lane. Some the ways in which you could elevate your alert level are:

Being alert is only a very general way to enhance memory. Even if you are someone with an excellent memory, you must try to be on alert the entire day. Being alert involves not just observing everything that comes your way but also registering them in your mental radar to come back to later when it comes up. A student must always be on red alert regarding things that might matter to his academic life.

Staying alert involves being attentive in classes, listening to every word the professor is uttering. It also includes staying updated on the recent developments in the field he is a student of. Many subjects are of the nature of changing all the time. They keep shifting their dynamics from day to day. Such subjects are usually branches of Science since every moment there is a new discovery made, a new theory written, a new element stumbled upon.

Meals

You may not realize it yet but skipping meals leads to a lot of complications for you. Especially if you are a student, your meals matter the most to you. You practically start your day with a meal, i.e. breakfast. The breakfast is the most important meal of your day as it provides you with the energy to drag through the day. It becomes all the more important for those pursuing academics, since they are always in the hurry to remember stuff. Food gives you the nutrients that help your memory not just pick things up fast, but also retain them for a long period of time. Meals should never be skipped in the rush of studying a lot.

A lot of students make the mistake of skipping meals in their hurry to finish their syllabus. Do not fall prey to the argument that if you skip meals and save time you will be able to study more. It is a gross misconception. When you skip meals, leave alone being able to study more, you tend to forget whatever you have mugged up so far.

Nutrition can be used to effectively to help the brain to combat symptoms associated with lack of focus and restlessness. Research shows that both diet and supplementation with minerals, multivitamins and other nutrients can work in a similar manner. For instance, supplementing with minerals daily has been found to be effective in vitamin-deficient people. However, do not specifically rely on supplements, as taking high amounts of minerals may be toxic for the body.

That said; supplementing with Omega-3 such as taking of fish oils may minimize the memory-related conditions in some children. In a research, it was found that administering about 1 gram of Omega-3 for about 3-6 months showed medium to strong effectiveness on ADHD condition. Other findings also suggest related results, especially in cases where Omega-3 fatty acids are incorporated with magnesium and zinc.

The following are nutritional tips that can help manage poor memory and attention deficit condition:

- ✓ Ensure to eat a diet rich in protein from breakfast, lunch, snacks and during dinner or as desert. Eating protein rich foods ensures a slow but steady release of dopamine, which help keep you motivated throughout the day. When you are motivated, you accommodate new information positively.

- ✓ Eat lesser simple carbohydrates, avoiding products such as white flour products, sugar, white rice, corn syrup, and potatoes without skin.

- ✓ Reach for more complex carbohydrates especially at night, which aids in better sleeping patterns. Such a diet should include tangerines, grapefruit, apples, kiwi, pears or oranges.

- ✓ Obtain more omega 3 fatty acids from fish such as tuna, salmon and cold-water white fish, olive oil, canola oil, Brazil nuts as well as walnuts.

- ✓ Restrict food rich in sugar, caffeine and artificial flavors since they area direct contributor of inability to grasp information.

- ✓ Eat enough calories as these are used to control amount of oxygen supplied to the brain. This will in turn improve the level of concentration and help you incorporate new information easily and effectively.

Read To Understand, Not Mug Up

Another common folly that students commit while preparing themselves for exams is that they tend to rot things up rather than understanding the concepts and the fundamentals of most subjects. Before you get down to mugging things, remember that this is a subject and a subject is not something that is to rot-learned. A subject has a history, a rich premise, an understanding that goes deeper than a few pages of published material. If you want to excel in studies, make sure that you get yourself familiar with the base of the subject you are trying to master. It helps a lot when you have grasped the reasoning and the history behind a particular subject. I am speaking from my personal experience here. The more familiar you get with the history of your subject, the better positioned you are to grasp the branching out theories that flow from it. It is only by going to the root of a tree rather than reaching out to the leaves, that you will be able to nurture a tree, Your education is the tree, the pages its leaves, and the history of it its roots. Go to the roots to study the tree.

Familiarity Breeds Memory

A major blunder that students worldwide do is that they start preparing for their exams a night before the scheduled date. I am personally guilty of the same blunder and hence, yet again I am speaking from experience. Allow yourself time to prepare for an exam. You may not realize it but the more time you spend with something, the better etched it remains in your head. Try recalling songs you listened to in your childhood. You would be surprised at how clearly you remember the tunes if not the exact lyrics. Why else do you think we can so clearly remember some of our fondest memories from our past? It is only because we spent enough time building those memories.

Grow familiar to your subjects. This is the most basic way to excel at your subject. Try to pick up your reading material and studying it while you are hanging out in your lawn in a sunny afternoon. This way you not only keep yourself engaged but also slowly but surely get familiar with something you are to encounter after a few months.

Of course, study material related to academics bore most students but try to think of them as leisurely activities and not a burden and then you will be good. Most tedious of all courses can be tackled well if sufficient time is spent studying them. When you are studying your reading material in your leisure hours, make sure you do not focus all your energy understanding every detail given there. You will most likely find it dull that way. Try speed-reading your subject while on leisure. This way you will find out that despite not getting what has been written, you will at least register the experience thereby creating a by default folder in your mind.

The very experience of failing to grasp a concept will create a memory in your mind that in turn will register itself.

Hence, even in failures you end up retaining something that is important to you. Grow familiar with your studies in order to create the perfect atmosphere for studying them with ease a night before.

Use Literary Devices

Over time, there have been invented a plethora of literary devices to help student gain mastery over education. These literally devices are each unique in their own ways. Not every student is perfect. Even the top scoring student has doubts and second thoughts of his own. Try chatting with someone who has scored good in some subject and you will discover that they took help of literary devices at some stage or the other. Some of the most used literary devices used worldwide are enlisted below:

Buzzwords

A buzzword is a word that triggers a train of chain of thoughts in your mind. You must have read a hundred scrolls regarding a particular topic and yet when it comes to the moment of performance nothing comes to your mind. However, there is always a bunch of such words that are so fundamental to the topic that their mere utterance or recalling even triggers you to recall the entire topic as you read it.

Allot buzzwords to separate topics. By doing so, you will realize that you have for each topic just one word to recall. Hence, with the help of just one word you will be able to write and memorize the knowledge contained in a hundred scrolls. Buzzwords are really helpful when it comes to retaining stuff that is lengthy in nature.

Learning

For example, imagine a law student having issues with recalling the punishment prescribed for murder, homicide and suicide. The word that connects these three offences is 'life' and somehow he is not able to recall what these three separate offences stand for. However, if he recalls just one word that is 'life', everything that he has read about these three offences comes rushing to his mind. This is how buzzwords help you recall things that are complicated and lengthy to remember.

Acronyms

Acronyms are nothing but new words formed from a group of words. An acronym is usually a fun thing to remember. The ordinary set of words may not make sense to you but when converted into an acronym, they somehow relate to the main subject and are fun to say out loud. This way it is ensured that you enjoy memorizing things in the best way possible.

For instance, a student having problems with recalling the nine planets of the solar system could easily take help of the following acronym

My Very Educated Mother Just Showed Us Nine Planets

Let us understand how acronyms work. Take the first letter of each word of the above sentence. Mercury, Venus, Earth, Mars, Jupiter, Saturn, Uranus, Neptune and Pluto are the nine planets whose names can be inferred by simply recalling a mere sentence.

Acrostics

The difference between an acronym and an acrostic is that while in the former, a sentence is formed; in acrostics, a word is formed. The basic underlying principle of both of the devices is the same, i.e. to recall the original words from fun words or letters. Let me illustrate how an acrostic works:

You must have studied physics at some point of time in your life. If you are a student, you must have come across the phenomena of splitting of light into its constituent colors. These colors are seven in number and often prove headache to most students. However, a simple acrostic called Vibgyor could be recalled in order to exactly spell out all the colors in the rainbow. Violet, Indigo, Blue, green, yellow, orange and red are the seven primary colors that can be seen in a rainbow and recalling them has been made easy by a mere word.

Method of Loci

Historians who were also public speakers first used the famous Method of Loci. It was a common hindrance for such people when they would not exactly remember what teachings they were about to impart to the onlookers. Having embarrassed themselves scores of times, they devised a method to remember exactly how they experienced it.

The Method of Loci is a very practical way to remember things. Here is how it works. Imagine walking from your college to your home. You will come across the grocery store, the neighbor's house, the local park and various other such landmarks while you are on your way. Now, repeat this every day when you actually walk back from college to home.

Having successfully implanted this route inside your mind, it is now a child's play for you to remember things. All you have to do next is associate each landmark with something you have to remember for your exams. For example, you could associate your neighbor's house with the Pythagoras theorem because of the shape and placement of his house.

Method of Loci is a beautiful way to not just recall stuff that you tend to forget but also retain them for your life as this is based on something you have personally experienced and devised. The Method of Loci as has been mentioned is entered around one's personal experiences in life and is bound to vary from person to person. Every person has his or her own forms of executing the method. However, the method has been proved to have worked in most cases and has seen few instances of failures.

Parts

A major mistake most students make while studying for exams is that they try to take in everything all at once. You need to grasp the concepts of taking in parts. When you divide your studies into compartments and sections, each to be studied at different time and according to varying moods, you are bound to achieve success.

No one has ever succeeded at studying and retaining everything at once. Give your mind some time to recover from the intense studying you have done in the past some hours. Take constant breaks so as to allow your memory to first register everything that went into it. Let the windows of your mind and memory stay open for a while before diving to study further.

Rhymes and Rhythms

Are you familiar with ancient folklores about famous mythological verses like the Ramayana and the Mahabharata? One story says that the sages who told the world about these stories sang them. Now, Mahabharata

Learning

happens to be one of the longest stories the world has ever heard, with its verses going as long as eighteen thousand pages. Do you know the secret behind how someone could just 'speak' the stories to masses? It was said that these sages simply sang these stories.

It has been scientifically proven that when you convert something into a song, with a set tune that does not change the next time you sing it, it sticks with you. Tunes have a certain retaining power to them. When you repeat tunes, they are bound to stay back in your head and with enough practice; they come naturally to you when you try to recall something. Convert your study material that is proving difficult for you, into songs and rhymes.

Association

A good mnemonic device, though not per se, is association. You cannot study in isolation, i.e. when you study you cannot separate its parts into dull individual bits and hope to remember them all in the end. Everything that you read is connected within itself. For example, if you are reading about the French Revolution then you are bound to remember something about the fall of the Berlin Wall. This is called the technique of association. One part is always connected in this way or that to the others.

Flash cards

These are simple cards, which you write short notes when studying to help you remember the details at a later time. You can make them yourself how you want or buy them from professionals. These tips can help you use flash cards effectively to boost memory and learn faster:

- Try not to store too much information on a single card.

Learning

- You can use both sides of the cards where necessary

- Use different colors of flash cards to convey different nature of information, like resentful to go on yellow or red cards, or white for neutral words.

- Try to decorate the cards to make the information written on it memorable, like sticking a piece of magazine on top.

- Have your flash cards with you when studying. Write down specific information that you come across when you are studying that you want to remember.

- When you are through studying, make sure you have your cards with you at all time and go through them when you are free.

- When reviewing your cards, shuffle them up so that you remember all information regardless of the order in which the cards are arranged.

- During your free time, revisit these notes to keep the information you have learnt fresh in your brain. Going through your notes repeatedly to refresh your memory helps you to understand things better.

Learning

Chapter 5: Imagination And Memory

Welcome to the fourth and the final section on memory. You have learned everything there is to know about memory enhancement. You are now equipped to excel at your studies. You are less likely to forget why you came all the way to the kitchen to open the fridge door. You are technically well versed with the art of memory improvement. Yet, there is something missing in all this. Is applying mnemonic devices enough? There is definitely something more to memory development than mere acronyms and association formations.

No sane man has ever disputed the power of imagination. A canon can kill people, but imagination can build people. Imagination has the power to transcend boundaries of any nature and fly like an eagle in the open sky. When you imagine, you are liberated and there are no sort of restrictions put on you. Imagination gives you the power to open your minds to dimensions never explored before. But why are we talking about imagination in a book revolving around memory improvement? Let us find out.

Imagination is an exercise that is wholly personal to you. What you imagine is radically different from what the other person does. Because of how complex human mind is, imagination has no fetters put on it. You cannot draw lines around a mind and ask it to imagine within those boundaries. Imagining is hence a never ending process and a very personal one.

Your imagination of a perfect holiday might fundamentally differ from your partner's. The destination may be the same, and the timing, but it is the beauty of imagination to differ despite the premise being the same. This is what

Learning

happens when you imagine. You create images inside your mind that are not just personal but also unique to you. You have a set mental image of what you think and that separates your imagination from those of others. As a result, no single person's images are the same as that of the others. This leads to your images standing out in a crowd.

A mere recollection leads to the rushing of everything you had imagined related to a particular topic. Hence, it is natural that whatever you imagine remains etched inside your mind forever. Though it is true that you rarely share your imagination with others, you keep sharing it with your own self. That way, you keep thinking of it in a loop thereby cementing its picture inside your memory.

Students get to only read what is there in their syllabus. Except for lab work and associated Google images, when students start imagining with the help of the written words, they start creating a series of mental images that stay with them whenever they stop studying. Imagination hence leads to the strengthening up of a person's memory with time.

For instance, Albus read about the Indian struggle for freedom from a school prescribed book, and so did Fred. Albus created the image of a large rally crying out for freedom from its British rulers but when Fred read it, he imagined a large number of leaders assembling together in front of the parliament and offering a peace treaty for freedom. Words will remain the same; the images will differ. This is how imagination helps create personal experiences of studying, thereby facilitating each student differently. Imagination is a tool that has been long ignored in the era of new technology.

Let me give you another example of how imagination is important for a good memory. In the good old days of

Learning

Graham bell telephones, people would maintain telephone logs where they would write down the numbers of every contact they had. They would have to manually dial the numbers after having looked them up from this log. After having looked at the numbers for a certain period of time, they would start associating the numbers with how they were written. Maybe a scribble at the top of the page helped them remember a specific contact. The handwriting with which the number was written might also lead them to imagine the person it belongs to in a specific way.

The human mind works in peculiar ways and association by imagination is one of them. However today, we have smartphones that simply save numbers in the form of people's names. This form of saving numbers has led to most us being unable to recall numbers of even someone close to us, for example our parents or our spouse.

The lack of imagination in today's world is a major reason for people having bad memories. When you lack the creativity to think of an entity in ways better than it has been presented to you, you tend to see beyond the mundane and the ordinary. Try to make things extraordinary and interesting so that you can easily remember them. Do not look at a tree and go "oh look, a tree"; try imagining it as a freak monster from one of the fairy tales you read as a kid; you will remember the tree better the next time walk by it.

Spread the wings of imagination to the sphere of academics and you will realize that the most boring of mathematical equations are fun when put in a lighter perspective. It is upon you to make sure that things do not remain the way they are. Play with studies. Tweak the texts. Change the textbooks' words to fit your imagination without changing the fundamentals. Be a bit creative with whatever you are studying. Do not be monotonous while making notes in the class. Use differently colored pens to illustrate your moods while writing. When you perform such crazy tips, you will notice changes in your attitude towards studies.

What used to be a major pain your rear before is now a relief and a major attraction. You no longer have to suffer in academics, and even before you realize it you will have excelled in academics all the while having fun at it.

The more you imagine, the better you memory becomes. It is by imagination by you will be able to associate one entity with another. Imagination authorizes you to create any image you want and associate it with anything you want to recall later.

I personally know of public speakers that would have stage frights right a minute before their speeches. However, when they get on the stage they speak as fluently as any other good orator. Their secret, as I later discovered, was their imaginative capacities. Even when you are in front of a huge crowd and you are supposed to speak on a subject, you can always imagine the crowd to be an association of jungle animals who have no idea about what you are rambling. Such a funny image will not only lighten you up but also give you the self confidence to speak based on the casual assumption you just made about the crowd being a bunch of illiterate buffoons.

Remember, how you memorize things that matter to you is entirely in your hands. This book can only suggest and direct you towards generalized and commonly used forms of memory enhancement techniques but in the end, it all comes down to how you apply the same.

Imagination is a powerful memory tool. You imagine breaking away from the dull set notions prescribed by others. But you also end up creating an entire world all by yourself. Exactly how a parent never forgets to feed his

Learning

child, you are not likely to forget this world because it is your personal creation; something you made when you felt like thinking better, brighter and extraordinary.

Chapter 6: Ask And You Shall Learn

Actors have got to be some of the most underestimated bunch of talented people on earth. It's a common misconception that actors aren't as intelligent or mentally capable as say, accountants or computer programmers, to say the least. Maybe it's because what they do seems to be too easy in contrast to the amount of money they earn.

First off, not all actors earn tons of money. Those that do are just the top 5% or 1%. Most other actors do just fine while some are even struggling. But that's not the important misconception to correct.

The misconception that actors aren't the sharpest tools in the shed isn't just baseless – it's totally wrong! Being able to deliver lines, especially for live performances such as theater plays, doesn't just require memorizing thousands of words but also learning how to properly express those words in terms of tone, body language and even timing! Now I don't know about you but that doesn't sound like it's a very menial task to me!

Most people think that actors and actresses merely "memorize" all their lines by simply rehearsing them. In this case, most people are wrong. According to psychologist Helga Noice, many actors don't learn lines by trying to concentrate on their scripts' actual words but on things that run deeper: the context of the scene, what is really meant and their characters' persona and motivations.

That isn't to say that memorizing is worthless and should be thrown out as a learning technique. No, it still has its place in terms of learning but in order to be able to really learn something much deeper, you can go deeper into what

Learning

it is you're trying to learn by explaining why it is the way it is.

What do I mean by this? Let's take the acting example from earlier. Suppose you're playing the role of a hostage taker, who's doing it because he feels he was given really poor cards to play life with. He feels the government and society in general have conspired against him as within the last 3 months alone, he lost his job, his wife and his kids to retrenchment, divorce and court ruling, respectively.

To be able to learn how to play the role exceedingly well, try explaining why the hostage taker is doing what he's doing. To be able to do this, you'll need to ask questions concerning what you're trying to learn. In this case, put yourself in his shoes and see how you'd feel if the same thing happened to you. If you can't, recall an incident in the past where you felt like you were treated by life, fate or society in general unfairly.

When you're able to do that, you'll be able to explain away why the hostage taker is really doing what he's doing and in the process, put yourself in the best position to play the role. You learn how to play the part as if you really were the hostage taker.

This method of learning how to play roles isn't just "showbiz" stuff – it's actually based on a practical learning technique that can be used to learn just about anything – faster and better. This technique is referred to as elaborative processing or investigation. In this technique, you relate the information to other relevant and associated information and facts.

In one study, a group of participants were instructed to learn some words by trying to explain or answer one of 3 questions. The first 2 questions were about the word itself while the 3rd question related the word in question to another word or idea. Guess which answered question led to the most significant ability to recall words? You guessed it right (I guessing you did) – the 3rd question, which explained what the word is particularly by relating it to some other familiar idea or word, which was more meaning-based and elaborative compared to the 2 other questions.

There was another study where the participants were asked to learn sentences this time. In this experiment, they learned the sentences by either studying the sentence itself or by elaborating or expanding on it with an explanation or investigation as to why the sentence was so. For example, the sentence is "Luke Skywalker was distraught." versus the sentence "Luke Skywalker was distraught because he found out who his true father was...Darth Vader!", the latter type of sentence led to improved memory and higher sentence recall. This seems to suggest that more cognitive effort can increase one's ability to learn something really well.

In yet another study, this time on the different ways of preparing for school tests, participants of the study were split into two groups. The first one were asked questions – the answers to which were the topics they'll be reading – before studying a particular written material. The other group was merely asked to study the written material. The study's results revealed that retention and recall of the studied texts improved significantly through elaborative processing or investigation, e.g., answering related questions prior to studying a certain topic.

Elaborative processing or investigation (explaining) is a good way to learn things to the extent that you'll be able to learn a particular material whether or not you actually try. In another study, two groups of people were asked to apply elaborative processing or investigation on a piece of text – one group were required to learn it while the other was merely asked to apply the learning technique. The researchers who conducted the study discovered no significant difference in the learning results for both groups, i.e., learning intention plays a minimal role in learning effectively compared to learning method.

Chapter 7: Self-Explanation

As a learning technique, self-explanation was observed to be particularly useful for kindergarten students as well as students who are trying to learn geometric theorems and algebraic formulas. Much like the elaborative technique you learned earlier, much of this technique's strength lies in its simplicity.

This is a learning technique that's best utilized for learning abstract materials. Under this technique, you explain a new fact or information by trying to connect it to other known ones. You also learn something new by explaining the steps necessary for solving a problem and justifying choices made to solve such problems. This technique was determined to be more effective at improving one's learning abilities when applied during the learning phase itself as opposed to after.

Basically, the self-explanation technique will require you to explain how you thought about something instead of just thinking of that something as a concept or a fact. Take for example, learning the financial concept of compound interest. A good way of learning this is asking yourself how the concept of compounding interest is related to something more familiar, like how a small snowball rolls downward to become a ginormous one in movies or cartoon shows. Or you can also explain the mathematical or logical steps involved in solving problems of compounding interest.

Some studies suggest that self-explanation is especially beneficial for learning how to solve puzzles that require logical thinking and reasoning. It was also found that students who utilized the self-explanation learning technique also exhibited better information recall, ability to solve problems and ability to apply the new things

Learning

learned to new content. In fact, there is reasonable basis for believing that this technique can be successfully utilized in practically any area of learning.

You can utilize this technique for your own learning by asking yourself things about how you processed the learning and not necessarily the learning content itself. A good question to ask, for example, is "How does my new learning relate to what I already know?" Incidentally, the best way to implement this in terms of self-learning is to ask questions whose answers are not yet known to you or aren't easily accessible, to train yourself in the art of asking good questions and to master the skill of explaining well.

Chapter 8: Summarization

Not to be confused with paraphrasing, which is merely changing a sentence or two into something that's about the same word content, summarizing is the process of condensing a resource material into fewer number of words. For example, you can summarize a paragraph into one or two sentences only or bring down ten pages worth of material into just one or two paragraphs. Summarizing gives you much leeway in terms of how to condense learning materials depending on your need or goal.

Summarizing is one of the best learning strategies or techniques because it forces you to:

- Spend quality time with the material you want to condense
- Deeply think about and study the material you want to condense and to segregate the important parts from those that aren't; and
- Rephrase or rewrite the main ideas or points you qualified as important in your own words.

All these things you're forced to do to summarize learning materials enhance your ability to learn them because:

- Spending time with your learning materials have a significant contribution to your learning them;
- Processing the relative importance of the points covered in your learning materials trains you to think critically and analyze; and
- Rephrasing or rewriting the materials you studied improves your ability to retain and understand them.

Learning

In particular, rephrasing or rewriting the learning materials in your own words can help accelerate your learning because it forces you to:

- Break down your learning materials further into simpler and more understandable bits;
- Focus your attention on what really matters; and
- Filter out the unnecessary information, points, ideas and examples in order to condense them.

These three activities are important especially in today's information overloaded world, which continues to be even more overloaded by the day. As too much chefs can spoil the broth, too much information can make us go crazy! Summarizing, therefore, helps us to not just identify and learn the relevant points and ideas but also to keep our sanity!

How To Summarize

Summarizing involves 3 key steps:

- Retention of key or important points or ideas;
- Omission of those that aren't; and
- Condense the material by trimming away less important stuff like narratives, descriptions, details and examples.

The degree of condensation varies between summaries, which depends on the amount of available information and the purpose for the summary, e.g., information abstract, study guide, future reference or mental exercise for remembering or retaining the key lessons of what you just read. Some summaries condense material to about 25% of the original content while others do so to as low as 5% of

Learning

the original! As a general guideline, the greater the content of the learning material, the more you should condense it. Why? Condensing a material of 10 pages down to 20% means summarizing it to just 2 pages, which is practical but doing the same (20%) to a 100-page material means cutting it down to a "mere" 20 pages, which is too much for a summary! <u>Keep in mind that the secret to summarizing as a good learning strategy is its brevity and condensation of ideas into the important ones only.</u>

An important part of summarizing is being able to ask good questions, which include:

- Why am I summarizing this material?
- What are this material's key points and ideas?
- What is the material's main point?
- Which of these points and ideas can be discarded or omitted?
- Which of these data, examples and descriptions can be further condensed for retention and which need to be thrown away?

Practical Tips For Using Summaries To Accelerate Learning

As mentioned earlier, we live in a world that's already – and continues to be – overloaded with information, which requires that we be able to quickly and effectively sift what's important or relevant from those that aren't. Here are some ways to help you cut through the much of the information fat of the learning materials you encounter for faster and better learning:

 If there are available summaries for the learning material, read them prior to reading the whole material. Aside from the possibility of discovering that such summary may be all that you need, you'll also have a better idea of which ideas and key points to consider within the material. In fact, you may be in a better position to understand individual points and ideas in the material if you already saw the whole picture via the summary.

- Utilize summary "shortcuts" such as paragraph or section headings, first sentences of a paragraph or the last sentence or two of the same, from which you can summarize the whole paragraph or section.

Learning

Chapter 9: Study Cycling

Often times, we think that learning techniques and strategies are simply all about, well, trying to learn! But as with other important areas of our lives, learning things also have optimal times, which can help accelerate or maximize our learning success if utilized properly.

One of the ways to practice this technique is to find out what our individual alertness factors are:

- When are you most alert, awake and able to focus and concentrate – night, noon or morning?

- How long can you focus or concentrate on a particular material or subject before such focus and concentration breaks and require you to take a break?

- What practices help you to concentrate and focus best?

To the extent that you are aware of when are you most productive in terms of learning is the extent you can effectively plan, schedule and cycle your studying or learning for maximum absorption and comprehension. Some things to consider in doing so include:

- Study materials that are most challenging during your "peak" learning times and the least challenging ones at any other time. If for example, you're not too good in math-related subjects and your peak learning time is usually late afternoon, then study math-related subjects on late afternoons.

- Incorporate the Pomodoro technique in your studying to help you keep optimal focus and mental freshness. The Pomodoro technique requires you to work or study for 25 minutes straight and resting for 5 minutes, which constitutes a Pomodoro cycle. This helps keep your mind fresh and prevents it from fatiguing too soon, thereby extending your mental productivity. You should be disciplined enough to rest at the end of each 25 minute work/study period even if you feel you're still good to go. Don't wait to be tired before taking a break so you can extend your peak mental performance time. After 4 cycles, take a 10-minute break instead of just 5 minutes and resume regular Pomodoro cycles.

Learning

Chapter 10: Keyword Mnemonic

When you walk into any bookshop, you'll find many self-help books that encourage using mnemonics as a memory improvement technique. Mnemonics is a study technique that utilizes just about anything that can help you remember or recall just about, well, anything. One way of doing this is by assigning images to certain information you want to learn or memorize. Let's try something fun that will help you see just how powerful mnemonics can be in terms of accelerating your learning process.

Let's try to learn the alphabet backwards: Z Y X W V U T S R Q P O N M L K J I H G F E D C B A. You could do your best by simply memorizing the whole thing, which may seem a bit daunting at first. Rightly so because you're probably looking at the reverse alphabet as a whole and thinking to yourself how on earth will you be able to memorize all of it in one fell swoop? I'm actually hoping you felt that way so that you'll be able to appreciate the following mnemonic techniques better, which can help you memorize the whole thing in 5 minutes or less.

Chunking

Chunking means grouping several of the letters into more manageable chunks of, say, 3 to 4 letters. It's no different from having to cut your favorite fillet mignon into smaller pieces before eating them as swallowing the whole thing can be fatal. Or like the way telephone numbers – especially those with area codes – are chunked together. Chunking the reverse alphabet would look like this:

ZYXW VUTS RQP ONM LKJ IHG FED CBA

Graphics

There's much truth to the saying that a picture paints a thousand words. Our minds think in pictures and can process them faster, particularly attaching your short-term memory, which in this case is studying the alphabet backwards, to an already existing idea or mental peg in your long-term memory. Simply put, learning in pictures is easier.

So how do you use graphics? Associate each of the letters with a picture in your mind – the crazier the better. Why? The crazier it is, the more memorable it becomes and the better your mind is able to retain it. For example, you can associate an electric guitar-wailing zebra to the letter Z. How's that for crazy huh? Do the same for all the other letters and see if you don't memorize the whole thing better and faster.

Learning Passwords

You can use mnemonics to assign passwords that are very hard for hackers to figure out but easy for you to remember. You can think of key sentences and use the first letters of each word as a mnemonic cue for your password.

- I Love My Wife Very Much = ilmvm or 1LMWVM

- My Dog's Name Is Barkley = mdn1b

- Psalms Is My Favorite Book In The Bible = pimfbitb

Learning

Chapter 11: Idea Mapping

This learning technique, also known as mind mapping, is an creative thinking or outlining method for putting ideas on paper. Compared to simple outlining, idea mapping is much better because for one, it isn't linear. As such, ideas can organically be mapped and grow because many of them don't follow a straight line anyway. What this means is ideas can flow back and forth while still being developed and branch out instead of being like ducks in a row.

Another advantage idea mapping has over simple outlining is that it allows for ideas or points to be connected to not just one other idea but several. You can connect them to others that precede or succeed it. You don't limit them in this sense.

A third advantage it has is that it's visual and spatial, which allows you to more quickly and better see the whole picture and the relationships of ideas with one another. You can easily see in just one glance, which ideas are more important and which ones are the least important, enabling you to focus better.

Lastly, an idea map is superior to simple outlines because it makes adding new information and relating them to what's already on the map much easier. You don't have to rewrite the whole thing – you can just draw another connecting arrow or line and write the idea.

There are many kinds of idea maps but there are two that stand out as among the most common and popular: the Cloud-Circle-Flowchart (CCF) and Tree Branch (TB).

Cloud-Circle-Flowchart Idea Map

In a CCF idea map, the main point or idea (also referred to as Level 1) is written at the center of the paper, with a cloud drawn around the idea. It's important for the sake of efficiency to write the idea first before drawing the shape because doing otherwise run the risk of the idea not being able to fit inside the shape, which can make your idea map look ugly and may force you to redo the whole thing.

Supporting ideas are written after the Level 1 or main idea/point and a shape is drawn around them as well. In order to illustrate its relationship to the main or other ideas, connecting arrows are drawn from the bigger idea to the smaller idea. Lower level ideas are also written, drawn a shape and given connecting arrows to other bigger, equally important or sub-ordinate ideas as well.

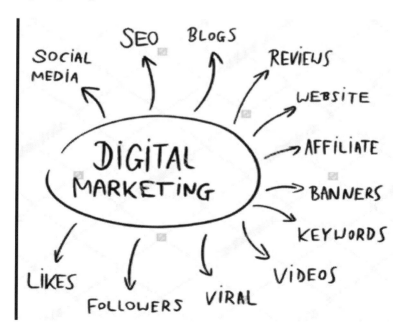

Learning

Tree Branch Idea Map

This alternative idea map is one that provides similar benefits as the CCF style but with an added benefit of being able to create sub-levels that can be visualized easier. In particular, this can be very useful if you have multiple sub-levels, e.g., main-sub-sub^2-sub^3 and so forth.

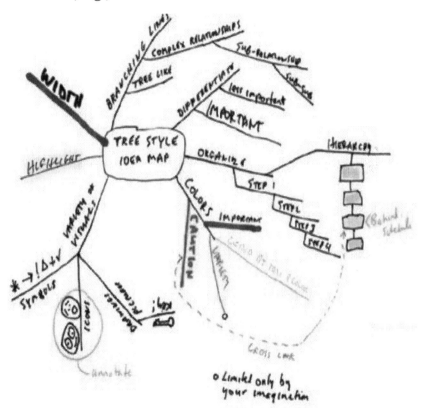

Idea Mapping Benefits

Aside from the superior points of idea mapping over simple outlining, here are other important benefits of using idea mapping as a learning technique:

- You can integrate complex ideas better by being able to add and connect ideas to any other idea or ideas;

- You can organically grow your sets of ideas and points by being able to add new points and ideas in seemingly random order without affecting the hierarchal and established relationships already established among the existing points and ideas;

- You can incorporate diagrams and pictures and connect them using links; and

- Because idea maps present ideas and points in a seemingly picturesque manner, your mind is able to better absorb and learn the material because the mind thinks better in pictures.

There are many free idea mapping software and applications that are available over the Internet for easier creation of such. However, doing it manually – at least in the beginning – can help you use such programs more efficiently. It's also worth noting that the physical act of writing down your ideas can help you learn ideas much better. You may want to use colored markers or pens and draw different shapes in different colors and sizes too. You can also emphasize more important ideas by making their shape's outline thicker or their letters bolder.

Learning

Here are more tips on how to manually create a good idea map:

- Our minds think better wider than taller and as such, it's a better idea to use a landscape orientation for your idea map's paper;

- As mentioned earlier, it's better to write the idea or point down first before drawing the shape to avoid making mistakes, i.e., ideas unable to fit within shapes;

- Write the highest level or main idea at the center of the paper; and

- Limit your ideas' words to a few words or a very short phrase in order to ensure that your map fits in the paper.

Chapter 12: How Idea Mapping Can Be Useful in Learning

Mind mapping is an easy way of simplifying the writing process and aids in doing away with unnecessary information, as you only capture the important facts. A mind map is a better way of note taking bearing in mind that each mind map fits in a single page. From the map, it's easier to note the connections, relationships and hierarchies at a glance. Let's see how idea mapping can help you in your day to day life to improve your learning and productivity:

Memorization

A number of times, note taking can be a struggle for many learners interested in memorizing book materials or notes. Taking notes even tends to result in an overflow of ink in every corner and margin on the page to some children. Mind mapping can help a lot in memorizing book materials and notes, and organize notes in a fun and easy way. With mind mapping, your thoughts can flow faster and recall process is simplified.

You can adopt mind mapping as a way of memorizing data or information, ranging from vocabularies of a second language to the technical and physical concepts. Mind mapping can help in utilizing the cortical skills and helps activate the brain at all levels. This role of mind maps makes the brain alert and skillful in remembering. The best thing about mind mapping technique is that they make the brain interested in revisiting them, thus facilitating the chances of spontaneous recall.

Learning

Assuming you want to memorize a course based on any topic, how can you use mind mapping for this? Follow these steps:

1. Begin by writing the main topic at the centre of a blank piece of paper. You need to focus on getting started without going to the extremes. For instance, a mind map on "American History" would rather be very lengthy and complicated. You can however choose to write "Luther King" at the center of the paper, and then draw a circle around the name.

2. From here, draw lines to other key concepts. Try to think of these lines as the main conveyance to the vital landmarks that you understand about the central idea. Decide on what you need to remember about the person and his contribution to American History.

3. Refer to your book and identify the major ideas you need to explore. As you get the information concerning a particular branch, think of a 2-3 words keywords to jot down under each topic.

4. Make the mind map work for you by trying to review the stored information from your map. Try to memorize parts of your mind map, and even recreate the map on a blank paper from scratch especially before taking an exam. Also, you can create flash cards from the main facts that are connected to a vital concept. Alternatively, you can quickly review the mind map you've just drawn.

Whenever you are studying a book or notes and need to memorize whatever you learn, make a mind map to depict the facts, dates, or lists. You can easily make physical associations between concepts and ideas by interacting with materials both visually and mentally. Thus, you can prioritize information into landmarks with precise supporting information, to help you recall the main concept more easily.

Boosting Creativity

One way to effortlessly boost your creativity levels is by learning to design good mind maps and use them for note taking, brainstorming, scheduling tasks, and assessing themselves. Doing this can boost your creativity and help you understand complicated lessons or ideas in day to day life. Furthermore, mind maps can further motivate you to get used to complicated assignments by use of images, colors, and visually appealing maps.

As you boost your creativity, you can easily assess yourself. A mind map can be effective in measuring your abilities based on your interaction with fellow learners, employees or other persons. From this assessment, you can set better goals that can be achieved within the set duration, as you boost and meet your day-to-day objectives.

Note taking

The traditional method of note taking involves the linear note taking to record important information, where you simply write down specific points as they are outlined. However, you can get more creative by adapting mind mapping to improve note-taking process. Likewise, majority of speakers or communication officials do not give information in a complete linear format. Instead, they seem to jump around and briefly present additional information to business ideas or research topics known or addressed previously.

Learning

Revising

Mind mapping can help a student revise their lessons and exam materials to recall everything covered in class. Each time a learner examines a map, it's easier to memorize the information on it to a larger extent. When you work more on the map such as by adding more pictures, colors, or details, this boosts the understanding of the map contents even further. Likewise, while studying exam materials, mind maps help you recall all details as studied in the classroom.

When revising, try to make short notes through a mind map to record the keywords, starting from the main topic to the branches, or sub-topics. Ensure that the map is very colorful by involving much creativity creating the map, drawing the images as well as showing relationships. Based on the rules of mind mapping, you can make a comprehensive mind map to help you read and pass exams. Try these simple steps:

1. Obtain a blank piece of paper, place it on landscape and then draw a circle, a square or an image that allows you to focus on the main topic in your map. Inside your central image, write the name of the topic or subject that you are studying. Make this as straight to the point as possible.

2. Continue with your study and come up with the substantial topics or related points that perfectly connect to your central theme. Then draw the branches from the central image, resembling the branches from a tree to connect the subtopics. Print your keywords on the branches while using block capitals in case you like that. You may also prefer to use geometric shapes to connect newer ideas, or sketch a little picture. Furthermore, you can use both, and why not?

Learning

3. Design your structure to mimic the keywords that you identified from the text. If you find some keywords or topics that lead you into making connections you didn't note initially, just continue. Create the relationships without being afraid of redrawing the map if it becomes messy. Also, make the pictures as funny, absurd or exaggerated as possible as your memory is more stimulated by vivid and funny images.

4. Start to branch off into smaller but related topics or sub-topics, ensuring you think very fast. Mind maps are supposed to work within an intense 5-7 minutes. Employ various colors of pen to bring out the connections between separate yet related topics. This also helps keep your mind stimulated. You are free to use pictures or symbols in case you find it more natural or practical. If bored at any stage, move on to create another branch.

5. Allow your thoughts and imagination to continue getting wild with each image. Mind maps need use of both images and colors that stimulate the right side of the brain. They should also be logical to stimulate the right side of the brain. When creating the images, don't get distracted by your poor images, as you don't have to be an artist to make a good map. All you require is a map that is understandable and comprehensive.

6. Continue repeating the above process of branches, colors and funny pictures, making each of the branches curved rather than a straight line. The brain is more trigged into action by curved lines.

Brainstorming

Mind mapping is an effective method and actually the most recommendable method of brainstorming. When you create a mind map, you activate your brain into action and thereby boost your creativity level. For instance, you may choose to draw a mind map before going to an examination room, before doing an essay or doing other challenging activity. Drawing the mind map enables you to retrieve the stored information from the brain and therefore create new ideas by association.

Those who developed brainstorming aimed to help generate many ideas as opposed to linear thinking that only results in a single solution. Actually, linear thinking only makes you to stop thinking! However, in brainstorming, a single idea you get will definitely lead to others to extend or modify the area. And where ideas tend to come in too fast, first note them down and then graft the tops to classify them later. So how can you do that without having to go overboard and stressing your mind?

1. Start by writing the areas of study in the center of a blank piece of paper.

2. Use colors, words, pictures and symbols to capture other topics, ideas, theories authors and other details concerning the topic. Position these at any position on your page, as you make free associations. Take care not to filter out ideas since everything is very important at this stage.

3. Now circle the key points or the ideas that you identified initially. Identify any gaps or missing information in your knowledge, and questions that may arise in the process.

4. Examine each of the items and see how the points relate to each other, and to the central topic. Use colors, arrows,

Learning

lines and words to map the relationships between the key points or ideas and link them together.

5. Find out the kind of connections that exist between points based on similarity, contrast, effects, or causes. Include these connections along with the linking lines.

6. Use your map as your guide or plan for your assignment, and then organize the items in a logical order to come up with a comprehensive structure for the assignment.

That said; what if you run out of ideas? In case you get out of ideas, reconnect by starting to draw in blank nodes. Since the human brain isn't intrigued by unfinished work, when you create "unfinished" or a blank node your brain is made to find effective ways of getting the work done. After gathering enough information as required, finally re-organize your topics or ideas until you obtain a completed and sensible structure.

There are various ways of recovering from lack of ideas at any point of brainstorming:

1. Get up and walk, or do anything that is very different just to come back after 30 minutes. Try to adopt repetitive activities that require less concentration, to allow the brain to relax and generate new ideas.

2. To some of your ideas or categories, just add blank topics. You will realize that your brain would with time work on ways of finalizing with the blanks. You can make the blank ideas anytime before going for a walk, to raise the chances of your subconscious mind being triggered to look for new ideas.

3. Come up with new random thoughts to facilitate creation of new words and associations, and then build your ideas from here. Don't worry on what the word or

thought is all about, as it's meant to save you from the worn pathways in the brain and make you think of new connections.

4. Find ways of boosting the existing solutions or other proposed ideas.

5. Reason whether there would be another viable solution and what would it be. This kind of self-questioning can trigger the brain to supply new ideas even when you thought there wasn't. After coming up with a new idea, your mind can then resume with flow of ideas.

6. Think on how other people would react if faced with the same situation. These people may be your competitors, your children, ancestors, workmates, or people from a different neighborhood or country.

7. To make your mind stimulated into a new line of thinking, seek for a definition and scope questions.

Summarizing content

Mind mapping can help a learner, manager or an employee to summarize books, essays, and articles all through the different academic levels. These materials may sometime become harder and more complicated especially if long and detailed, thus making memorization hard. When a learner takes notes when studying using mind mapping, idea mapping helps in memorizing the content under study.

One unique fact about mind maps is that they help you to break down complicated information into smaller and more understandable details. They help capture the key facts from a lengthy topic or idea and trigger the brain to understand and recall the content. Thus, mind maps are very important for revision of the content at a later date.

Presentations & reports

Mind maps can help a lot in analyzing information when doing or presenting a report. To make your presentation, just project your well-illustrated mind map onto a screen and then simply refer to whatever topic or fact you are addressing. In case you want to impress the audience, begin from an empty space and then progress to drawing a new map from scratch as you read your speech.

Though it may tend to be a harder process, you can prepare for your presentation by drawing the map beforehand say for 4-5 times. This can help in a big way when it comes to recalling it during the actual presentation. Whichever way you look at it, mind maps are there to facilitate recall.

When making mind maps for presentations follow these step by step tips:

1. Plan your presentation, and understand why you need to give it or why the audience needs to hear it.

Doing this help you to save your time and that for the audience. This is referred to as statement of purpose and is the most important part of any presentation. Just write it down as a single sentence, e.g. "purpose of my presentation is to educate the students on revising exams."

2. Use mind mapping to help you organize and present the information; by structuring your presentation in a very appealing manner.

A mind map allows a person to include an emotional attachment, such as by creating a branch referred to as 'feelings' or 'emotions'. This should allow you to explore the emotional features of your subject.

3. Make a build map that depicts the kind of presentation you have to make.

You may draw the mind maps a number of times, add attractive colors and symbols to ensure it sticks firmly into your mind. When done with drawing, your presentation is now memorized, and this can boost your confidence level while making the presentation.

4. Another creative way is drawing or displaying the map for the audience as you do the actual presentation. This can give your audience the visual structure in case they are to make notes. Ensure you feature as many pictures and colors to make the mind map visually interesting.

5. If you want your audience to recall whatever you are presenting, use different colors and keep the branches in different segments on your page. For instance, people can remember a topic just because it had "red coloring in the top left hand corner".

To-do lists

Most people try to manage time through 'To Do' list that involves making a list of tasks, classifying them based on priority and then working on the list. However, this method only suites simple tasks; and cannot be used for multiple tasks across different roles you need to do in a day. If working on day-to-day system, you may need to postpone all tasks to the next day, but if on an open-ended system, you cancel out those tasks done and then renumber the tasks. However, this method is somehow messy as it has no particular structure.

You can adopt idea maps to draw "To Do" lists to assist you remember the important task for the moment. You can sub-divide your to do list into groups such as "Homework",

Learning

"Class work" or "Current projects". For managers, you can easily design the extra curriculum activities line-up and to remind yourself about the personalities of different employees. Assessing employees' abilities can guide you when assigning urgent tasks, new projects, or business deals.

To make a mind map that can actually help you manage your time, try the following steps:

1. Get a piece of blank paper that is A-4 sized or larger, together with pink and yellow highlighters.

2. Begin by sketching a rectangle or circle in the middle of the page and write TO DO., together with the date of the week in the box or circle. Your labels may be 'To Do: 5-10 Jan 2016'. Ensure that you update the mind map daily.

3. Draw a branch arising from the center and then label it 'GOALS'. Think of a major grouping for your tasks.

4. Now draw a branch from the center to each of your major groupings, using a different colored pen. This may be referred to as 'Roles and Goals'.

5. List all tasks that you would aim to do in these areas; to act as sub branches that come from the main branches. Once done, you will obtain a pictorial representation of your tasks in one page.

5. Start to make a priority of your tasks. You need to track and manage the tasks to help you remain focused in the right thing at the best time. To do this, highlight the day's task in YELLOW, and number them in order of priority if possible.

6. To work on the mind map, follow the prioritized list based on the numbering until all tasks are completed.

Once done, highlight the tasks in PINK to constitute an orange branch that 'fades' into the back ground.

From here, you can easily track what has to be done and whatever has been completed, while preserving the history with sufficient clarity. You can apply your To Do list in various areas being a teacher, a parent, or a learner. As a teacher, you can have branches for your class presentation or for personal use.

Problem Solving And Decision Making

Mind mapping is a useful strategy for developing logical thinking by understanding the relationships between concepts and ideas. The flexible and friendly structure of mind maps assists learners to think better concerning ideas and concepts. The exposure to maps facilitates students to test information gathered to suite different scenarios. In so doing, mind maps enhance decision-making and problem solving by providing multiple options and solutions, which may not be realized in linear thinking.

The independent thinking brought by mind maps help students to generate multiple perspectives on problems, leading to better decision making. When a learner adopts mind maps to solve problems, the brain gains more clarity which helps get answers more easily. Thus as a learner, you can view problems as easy challenge or as a chance to show off your level of reactivity. Mind maps therefore prioritize the most vital element of your problem, i.e. focusing your mind.

To use a mind map to solve problems, follow these simple guidelines outlined below:

Learning

1. First make 2 separate mind maps, one outlining the problem while the other convenient solutions.

2. In the mind map for problems, make the initial problem as the central idea at the center of a blank piece of paper.

3. Add in as many branches based on the types and causes of the problem, illustrating every aspect using sub-branches.

4. After exploring a problem in this manner, you should find out why the problem occurred and what you can do to solve the problem.

Now make a second mind map with viable solutions following these steps:

1. Make 'Solutions' the main central idea.

2. Now add in the paths through which you can solve the problem being the main branches. You should involve as many techniques, colleagues, organizations or recourses that are beneficial, and make sub-branches to further get more details.

3. When using a mind map to solve problem, you will know that there are many solutions for just a single problem. Thus you ought to find out the option that is cost effective, time saver and very practical.

4. Now make a final branch that features the most recommendable solution or combination of solutions to solve a persistent problem. Draw sub-branches of the details revolving around the solution and then a way of implementing this.

Remember that you need to come up with many ideas to solve a challenge, and brainstorming can be the best method of exploring various potions.

Student Assessment and group projects

Idea mapping can also be applied by trainers or parents who want to monitor the progress of the learner or child in an effective but less tedious manner. Idea mapping works in two ways, to both the assessor alongside the learner to be assessed. For instance, mind maps can help a child to get motivation to express ideas more freely, which in turn act as a gauge to measure progress. In so doing, idea maps allow learners to recall information easily thus a positive outcome during assessment.

Mind maps can also help in simplifying the vital steps needed for a successful project work. Various people can adopt mind map to brainstorm together with their colleagues and get every member on the same reasoning level. This also helps in structuring the workload and sharing tasks.

Managing information

Mind mapping can really help in information management where you can collect the sources into a single map, design your chapter structure, and then organize the sources properly. For instance, let's assume that you are a researcher and need to create an academic paper. Depending on the length of the paper, you need to make a good structure for your sources and the actual content before you start to write. Thus, mind mapping can be made complete with color and diagrams to act as permanent record of courses or topics.

One way of managing information is having organized display of information, as it can be easily converted into a draft. That said; do you know you can use idea mapping essay writing? Mind mapping is a good strategy as it acts as a self-generated pre-writing activity. Learners just begin with a topic at the center of a blank page and then create a web of ideas from this. This is facilitated by the fact that associations result from developing and relating of ideas in the mind.

Another advantage of using mind mapping in essay writing is that they work well in their visual design, allowing them to realize the connection between ideas. This in turn helps them get motivated to group certain ideas as they go on writing. Mind maps are great when used in groups, since the group discussion aids in generation of ideas. Teamwork also makes a task livelier and very entertaining. However, sometimes you are alone at home without a chance of meeting other learners.

To mind map at the comfort of your house, you can follow the following steps to make an essay. All you need is a good point to start from and then pick up from there. Try out the following steps:

1. Start by brainstorming possible ideas or topics for your essay. You don't need to look for complicated ideas; just simple and random topics are okay.

2. Make various sub-topics that emphasize the main points. Make the structure for your essay by adding in new branches, which can develop the essay ideas even further.

3. Re-arrange the ideas ensuring you don't change or lose the content. Basically, a mind map should assist you analyze a variety of possibilities which is impossible to do in a linear format. Thus, you can play around the different ideas and organize the branches to get the best structure for essay.

4. Get motivating resources to help you develop the essay. You can incorporate these resources as audio

recordings, videos or links. A recommendable guideline is online resources before getting used to own ideas. Once done, ensure the essay represents your own line of thinking, your values and point of view.

5. Request for feedback from writing collaborators to help you create better articles. You can acquire an improved perspective on the topic you are writing, as a second opinion is always better.

6. Now add visual icons to the work already done, or if possible get an instructor to do the marking for you.

Remember that a good essay structure is a great choice for the target audience, thus ensure your ideas are catchy enough. Do this both at the start and ending of the essay, to impress the readers within the body of the article.

Chapter 13: Reading For Learning

We all know that reading is an imperative for learning in most cases, especially in school. Personally, I've learned so much since graduating through reading books and articles. Unlike going to classes at particular hours and having to adjust to the teaching pace, reading books and other materials offer the convenience of being able to learn at your convenient time and convenient pace. You don't adjust to the classes, the "classes" adjust to you.

Reading for optimal learning isn't as simple as, well, just reading. There is a systematic way of reading materials for accelerating your learning experience – the SQR3 technique. SQR3 stands for Survey, Question, Read, Recite and Review and is a good technique created to help improve reading recollection through different and repeated ways of engaging the material.

One key to memorizing something is repetition – the frequency of our engagement with something determines just how deep into our long-term memory it can sink. Some students go through their assigned readings two times to be familiarize themselves well with the material.

But as much as repetition helps us learn something, reading for optimal learning requires that such repetition also be systematic or methodical, i.e., there should be a method to the madness. One systematic reading technique was already discussed – summarizing. Another is the SQR3 technique. Let's take a closer look at the 5 important parts of this technique.

Survey

Learning

In this first step, you read the material simply by surveying it in order to get a general picture of overview. This step is also referred to as skimming or scanning. The reason behind this first step is that our minds prefer seeing the bigger picture in which to fit the individual parts together and see the general direction of the materials' authors for deeper learning and understanding. Having an insight of the sequence, arrangement and structure of reading materials give us the opportunity to create a mental framework from which we can build our learnings around.

If we know, for example, that a particular reading material's author is constructing a cause and effect reasoning, we can anticipate that he or she will discuss at least one cause followed by an enumeration of the effects of such cause.

It may be challenging to do this for relatively voluminous reading materials such as a monograph or a whole book. For these kinds of materials, it'll be beneficial to create a visual representation of the material's content. One useful tool – also discussed earlier – is the idea or mind map, which can help us monitor where we are mentally in terms of the discussion or argument flow. The idea map will also be particularly useful if the material is just borrowed and you need to return it soon – the diagram you created can help you find the ideas you're looking quickly and easily reacquire the discussion context.

So how do we survey reading materials? Well, it depends on the material. For books, here's how to do it:

- Read our book's blurbs (short descriptions written for purposes of promoting the book) showcased on its dust jacket or back cover.

Learning

- Check out its table of contents to get an idea of the topics that will be covered and how these are presented or organized.

- If available, go through the books chapter outlines, overview and objectives too.

- Quickly go through the book's pages, scanning its major headings.

- Check out the first chapter's major and sub headings as well as discussion at the end, if any.

- Check out the book's index to get an insight as to the topics the author discusses in the book.

For other reading materials, e.g., web pages, modules and articles, here are some helpful tips for surveying:

- Read the material's overview or abstract, if any.

- Check out its major and sub headings.

- If available, read the material's application, conclusion or summary at the end.

Question

Coming up with questions concerning your reading material makes you more curious, interested and pay more attention to it while reading it in order to answer them. You can come up with questions based on the material's graphics, pictures, chapters or headings and the idea map you made, if you have. Let's assume we'll read an archeological article on a recently discovered 20,000 year-old artifact. Here are good questions to ask to aid us in our reading:

- How will the author support his statement that the artifact is indeed that old?

- How will the author reply to potential criticisms or opposing theories?

- What are established dating techniques will he present to support his statement that the artifact is indeed that old?

- Have there been any developments, responses or issues on the subject since this material was published?

By coming up with questions, you'll be able to quickly pickup important points and ideas because you're already anticipating them.

Read

After skimming or surveying the book, the real reading begins. I highly discourage merely breezing through the reading material and just sitting back at this point in the reading technique. To the extent possible, highlight or mark important points and ideas of the reading material and as you do, re-read them for better retention.

Don't hesitate to write notes on your materials' margins. These notes may either be cross-references, examples (similar or opposing), objections, agreements, paraphrases or summaries. You can also draw tables or diagrams in your reading material's vacant spaces for making the ideas more graphic and easier to get.

If your reading material isn't yours or is a digital one, you can simply take down notes about the important points and ideas you come across within the material or copy important statements. Remember to cite the page number of what you note down for easier reference later on, if needed. You can also create an idea map or some other form of diagram on another medium to graphically represent the material. Once you're done, answer the questions you've written down earlier prior to reading the material.

Recite

The second of the 3 Rs refers to reproducing the key points and ideas gleaned from your reading the material. Reproducing can mean reciting them out loud, explaining these important points and ideas to someone else, summarizing by chapter, section or as a whole or paraphrasing key points and ideas.

A good way to recite these important points and ideas is by making an – you guessed it right – idea map! Other things you can create for optimal recitation are a list of frequently asked questions (including answers, of course), comments, summaries or outlines.

Why is reciting considered to be very important for learning? It's because reciting compels us to engage with our reading materials repetitively (good for reinforcing ideas), process important points and activate our visual and auditory channels for maximum learning.

Review

The last part of the SQR³ technique is reviewing. Here's how you do it:

- Go through your reading material's pages and read the headings (main and sub), the items you highlighted and the notes you wrote down.

Learning

- Go through the material's abstract or overview and any summaries you may have done. See if your notes and summaries are consistent with your reading material's points and ideas.

- Re-read your questions and answers.

- Pretend as if you're giving a speech to a bunch of people interested in your reading material by giving an impromptu commentary and summary of the material.

Raising The Bar

For continuous learning improvement through this technique, consider doing any of the following fun activities:

- Compose a poem, haiku or song, the words of which refer to your reading material's key points and ideas.

- Write a script for a play or movie scene wherein its actors discuss your material's key points and ideas.

- Make a PowerPoint presentation for the reading material you just covered.

Chapter 14: Speed Reading

Consider the volume of material you read every day, whether it's the daily newspaper, its online version, your favorite magazine or books both physical and electronic. Consider too the number of emails you read every day and despite that, the number of unread emails sitting around in your inbox, be it personal or work-related. Also, why not add into the mix the numerous data and reports that flood your desk – if you're a manager at work – that you not only need to read but to understand.

Whew, that's quite a load, isn't it?

Considering that reading is one of the primary ways to learn, we need to accept the fact that it's not practical to apply the SQR3 technique all the time. That's the ideal but let's face it – we live in fallen world that isn't perfect and at times, there's a need to read more material than there is available time. So what are we to do?

We need to read much faster – but effectively too.

Speed-reading is an important learning skill to acquire as it can help us cover more learning materials with less time. It's a great help in acquiring much knowledge that's needed to get ahead in today's very competitive world.

As mentioned earlier, SQR3 is the ideal and preferred reading technique for optimal learning. That being said, speed reading shouldn't be applied to reading materials that contain a great deal of important details, particularly legal documents. In such documents, missing out or misinterpreting just an iota of detail can prove to be very costly later on.

One of the reasons that most of us aren't able to read at optimal speeds is poor reading habits. There's good news and bad news about it, but let me start with the bad news so the good news really sounds good. The bad news is that such habits are so sly and deceitful that most of us hardly ever know we're guilty of them or that they're bad habits reading habits to begin with! The good news is that just like most insidious and inconspicuous villains in the movies, they can be overcome. And when we overcome them, we can significantly increase our reading speed and accelerate our learning.

Poor Reading Habit #1: Sub-Vocalization

The first reading habit that keeps us from reading at optimal speeds is sub-vocalization. This is our habit of saying each and every word we read mentally. Let me guess, that's how you're reading this e-book now, eh?

You may be wondering what the heck is wrong with reading every word mentally? At least I don't bother the person beside me. Here's the things: trying to keep pace with our mind's "voice" tends to slow down our reading. It's no different from reading texts verbally – word by word. It's because our minds can read significantly faster than our lips and hence, mentally "saying" them has the same mental reading effect as reading materials aloud.

How do we turn off that voice inside our heads? First thing is to acknowledge that we do sub-vocalize. We can't correct something that we don't acknowledge to be real. Upon doing that, we simply decide to "silence" that reading voice. No frills, no fuss and no magic voodoos needed. We just simply choose to read as fast as we mentally can, eschewing that reading voice inside our minds. In time and with practice, it becomes our new reading habit, albeit a good one.

Another approach to quitting the sub-vocalization habit is through reading in blocks of words. We'll look at how to do that in more detail later on.

Poor Reading Habit #2: Word Reading

The next poor reading habit that constricts our reading speed is reading each and every one of the words in our reading materials. What I'm trying to say is reading this text exactly – how – you – are – doing – now, - going – through – each – and – every – word.

We can't really blame ourselves now, can we? After all, we were all taught how to read in preschool by doing this – word for word. There's nothing wrong with that – at that age and stage. Unfortunately, no one was kind enough – or wise enough – to tell us to ditch the practice once we learned how to read. We carried this habit all the way up to this point in our lives and unfortunately for many others, to their graves. Consider this example that you'll read in 2 different ways:

- I;
- Will;
- Ride;
- My;
- Bicycle;
- All;
- The;
- Way;
- To;

- San; and
- Jose.

Now read the same word cluster like this:

I Will Ride My Bicycle All The Way To San Jose

Which of the two was easier to understand and faster to read? I rest my case.

Poor Reading Habit #3: Eye Motion

You may not be aware of it but the way we move our eyes when we read significantly affects our reading speed. One poor way of moving our eyes was the previous poor reading habit. The other one is reading each text line in one singular and continuous movement, unable to utilize peripheral vision for reading words at the start and end of each line of text.

People who are adept at speed-reading don't move their eyes this way. They read word blocks instead of individual words and by doing so, only move their eyes once or twice along each line of text instead of reading each and every word.

Poor Reading Habit #4: Regressing

This habit refers to our tendency to frequently go back to what we've already read – and this can significantly slow down our reading. Although doing this every once in a while can be helpful, particularly for complex ideas, doing this frequently isn't. Not only does it slow you down but that it breaks your reading momentum, which can give you a very challenging time in terms of getting the gist of your reading materials' structure and consequently, your ability to learn the materials. I highly discourage this habit but if you really need to go back to certain points in your reading material for learning's sake, do so sparingly.

One way to reduce your regression tendencies is to use an object like a pen (with caps on), your finger or an unsharpened pencil to mark your eyes' stopping points along each line of text you're reading. Doing this gives your eyes something to follow and overcome the poor reading habit of regression.

Poor Reading Habit #5: Being Distracted

Have you ever experienced reading something with either the TV or the radio on? How'd that work for you? Chances are, you weren't able to really absorb or learn that which you were reading, right? Even if for some mutant reason you were able to understand some of it, you know that you could've done better if you read without the TV or radio on.

Simply put, we need to optimize our reading environment if we want to be able to read effectively and fast. The best environment to do that is one that has the right temperature, adequate lighting and is silent. Such an environment will really help us focus on what we're reading.

Avoiding distractions is like dieting – it's simple but not necessarily easy. The primary reason for this is mental. Often times, we crave distractions and suffer separation anxiety when we get rid of them. C'mon – don't tell me you find it hard not to listen to One Direction or Metallica when reading? Remember, liars have long noses! The only

Learning

solution really is will power. As Nike always says – just do it!

One ray of hope is that on average, it only takes about 21 straight days of practice to break old habits and acquire better ones. So think of it as just a 3-week boot camp. After that, you'll find yourself asking "Why didn't I do this before?"

More than physical distractions, the more challenging ones to get rid of are mental ones. With physical distractions, we can simply set up our rooms or go to a place that's conducive for optimal reading but internal distractions tag along wherever we go! You'll need to wage constant battle for the next 3 weeks but after that, you'll find that it will no longer be a battle.

A simple but effective strategy to minimize such distractions in most cases is to take care of personal business before sitting down to read. Often times, it's those loose ends that distract us mentally, begging us to come hither and fix them! Procrastination is the primary reason for this habit and once again, the only solution here really is will power. Again, think 3-week boot camp.

How Fast (Or Slow) Do We Read?

For all our discussion on what speed-reading is and our poor reading habits that get in its way, we haven't really talked about the central theme of this chapter – reading speed. We won't be able to know if we're progressing in our attempts to read faster if we don't know how fast (or slow) we're actually reading. It's like the impossibility of staying within the speed limit at the Autobahn with a broken car speedometer.

To know your current reading speed, do this:

Learning

- Prior to reading, count your materials number of words, which should be much easier if you're utilizing a word-processor like Microsoft Word or Mac's Pages. But if your reading material is on paper, a good estimate would be to get the average number of words per line for the first 2 lines of text and multiply it by the total number of lines in your reading material.

- Read the whole material while timing yourself. As soon as you're finished, divide the material's total word count by total time it took you to finish reading – in seconds – and divide the resulting figure by 60. This is your estimated reading speed expressed in words per minute or WPM. At this point, you have now established your beginning or baseline reading speed from which you'll base your progress on.

- For convenience, there are many online speed-reading tests you can take to estimate your baseline reading speed. Just keep in mind that average reading speeds may differ between printed and electronic material. The important things is to be consistent. If you measured your baseline WPM online, continue measuring for progress online too. If your online reading speed increases, it follows that your printed one did so too.

Goal Setting

When trying to improve our reading speed, we need to set goals. Why? Without goals, we won't have any objective basis for establishing whether or not our efforts have succeeded or failed. It's no different from backing the car out of the driveway without any destination in mind. It will just be a waste of time and precious petrol.

When setting a good speed-reading goal, what is considered realistic? Here's a good guide (not a gold standard) as to average reading speeds:

- 200 to 250 WPM for children 12 years old and above;
- 300 WPM for college students;
- 450 WPM for college students who are skimming materials just for the main points;
- 600 to 700 WPM for college students searching for keywords in texts;

It's worth keeping in mind that the goal of speed-reading isn't to just "read" as many words as humanly possible within a given time frame. The real goal is to learn as much as possible within a given period of time, as measured in words read per minute. It's estimated that we can still comprehend as much as 75% of what we read up to 700 WPM and anything higher runs the risk of reduced learning.

A good goal to aim for are increments of 10% from the last most recent WPM. Remember, since the ultimate goal of speed-reading is to learn, you shouldn't be hurrying things up. Take your time and don't rush – unless of course someone's holding a gun to your head and being able to read at a certain speed can save your life. Otherwise, take baby steps and be realistic so that speed-reading can actually improve your learning.

Ready, Get Set, Speed!

Alright – now that we covered the basic principles and concerns of speed-reading and have identified a realistic goal, we'll look at how to actually speed-read.

Learning

Keep Your (Mental) Mouth Shut

Remember our discussion on the poor reading habit of sub-vocalization and how we said the only solution really is to zip it? One good way to "physically" shut our mental mouths up is by chewing gum as we read. Why is this such a brilliant, world-changing idea? Well, it's because chewing gum physically activates the muscles responsible for our being able to speak, which indirectly influence our tendency to sub-vocalize. If our physical mouth is busy chewing gum, it sends the signal to the brain that it can't mentally "speak" the written word. As such, we avoid sub-vocalizing. Cool, huh?

No gum around? No problem! Simply putting a finger or two on our lips should do the trick as it has the same effect of keeping our physical mouths from "reading" our materials as chewing gum, albeit in a slightly awkward manner.

Cover Operations

Another way to help us read faster is by covering up the texts or words that we've already read, which helps minimize the need for or the tendency to regress – another reading habit that slows down our ability to speed read.

One way to do this really well is by using an index card, which is what I personally do, to put a lid on the words I have already gone through. Keep in mind that this isn't supposed to be a permanent speed-reading crutch but more of a temporary training equipment, so to speak. As such, don't abuse it and over time, you should be able to ditch it.

Efficient Eye Movements

We may think that reading means having to move the eyes but the truth is, we read only when our eyes aren't moving. Reducing our eye movements' frequency per reading line can help us read and learn much faster.

It's been estimated that on average, we can read as far as 8 letters to the right of the point at which we fix our eyes and only 4 letters left of the same point. In terms of word count, this translated to about 4 words at most per stop or eye movement. With this, we can estimate our ideal eye movement frequency per line of X number words.

Here are some easy exercises to train your eyes to move less while reading:

- Place an index card on the line immediately above your text line of choice. Write an "X" on the index card's portion corresponding to the text lines first word.

- Place another "X" on the index card, this time on top of the 3rd word after the first "X" for challenging reading materials, after the 5th word for relatively easier reading materials or after the 7th word for simply skimming through materials' important points. Draw more "Xs" on the same index card line until you reach the end.

- Start reading as fast as you can by sliding down the index card with the "Xs". Read each text line by fixing your eyes on points on the text lines that fall under the "X" marks on your index card. Do the same for each line as you slide the index card down.

> Over time, your eyes will be trained to read with as few movements as possible.

Lastly, do focus on the current text line you're reading and please don't pay attention to those below and above it. Doing this helps maximize reading speed.

Speed Brain Training

As I said earlier, speed reading isn't done just for the sake of reading fast because the real reason for this is to understand and learn as much as possible within a given period of reading time. So more than simply training our eyes, we also need to train our brains for speed.

We can look to how runners train for marathons when it comes to speed-training our brains, particularly using the progressive overload principle. Progressive overloading means gradually building up reading speed and comprehension in increments that are just slightly faster than what we can currently understand. As our brains adapt to the next slightly faster level, we raise the bar yet again ever so slightly and repeat the process several times more until we achieve our desired speed. Doing it this way increases our chances for success while minimizing our risk for burnout and quitting.

So how can we do this in real terms? Here's how:

- Read a text line by moving a pencil from the beginning to the end of it. Say "one 1,000" at a very normal and relaxed speed and the pencil should reach the end of the line only by the time you finish saying it. This becomes your estimated baseline reading speed.
- Continue reading the other lines of text at the same speed. Never mind if at first, you find it challenging

to comprehend the words you're reading. Just focus on reading the other lines at the same speed for about 2 minutes.

- Stop to rest for about a minute then resume reading but this time, do it faster. The speed? You should be able to cover 2 lines of text in one relaxed and normal paced saying of "one 1,000". Continue reading the next lines at this pace for about 3 minutes.

- Do this exercise for 3 weeks – the average time to build new and kick old habits – and note the improvement in both reading speed and comprehension.

Skim Reading

Skim reading or skimming is another excellent way to build up our reading speed. The top benefit of practicing this is the ability to quickly get an understanding – however shallow – of a particular reading material. This can prove especially useful for extracting the main gist of newspaper feature or get the central details of any submitted reports, to name a few. This speed reading technique, however, isn't advisable for learning materials that involve a great amount of crucial details, as with the case of legal documents and job postings.

So what does it mean, in practical terms, to skim read? We start by simply reading the materials' chapter titles and main sections' headings and sub-headings. This is ideal for reading newspaper headlines or the table of contents of books and magazines. It's particularly useful to me in terms of deciding whether or not to buy a book or magazine within a limited amount of time.

We can read an article, section or chapter's first and last paragraphs, particularly their first and last few sentences, for a relatively deeper skim reading. This can also help us get a good idea of what their main ideas are.

When skimming, it's also helpful to circle words that we think are helpful for understanding the material. These words include proper nouns, unfamiliar words, words in different-styled fonts, repeated words and main points/ideas.

Visual Representations

Since a picture paints thousands of words and our minds think better in pictures, then it follows that looking at visual representations of reading materials' contents is a very effective way of skimming through their main points. This is one reason why most annual financial reports of large corporations incorporate nifty looking graphs and tables into their professionally written material. Simply looking at a pie chart, for example, immediately shows us what department accounts for most of the company's income for the year without using more words than what is needed to simply identify the departments.

Graphs can also come in handy for when it comes to skimming, particularly if we'd like to see a particular subject's performance over a span of time. Without even needing a whole paragraph, we can already learn that subject's multi-period performance just by looking at a graph.

Charts, pictures and diagrams allow us to skim and immediately get the main points of our reading materials without having to go through pages of high-faulting write-ups. Talk about efficient learning?

Learning

Just a friendly neighborhood advice – these visual representations, although effective, are only so up to a certain point. In particular, they're great for extracting main points or ideas but not for getting a deeper understanding of such. Learn to use them wisely for accelerated learning.

Learning

Chapter 15: Note Taking

One of the classic and most common strategies for accelerating learning that's often taken for granted is note taking. It's interesting to note that the mere act of taking notes — even if we don't review the notes afterwards — already increases our learning because doing so involves active listening, focusing attention on the topic, sifting through important and unimportant points and ideas, utilizing visual and auditory channels while writing and summarizing points and ideas. That shouldn't mean, however, that we shouldn't review the notes we wrote down. When we go through them afterwards, our learning is even more enhanced, especially if we process them further by summarizing them or making an abstract.

Although taking notes seem to be quite a simple and basic activity, we can do it in a way that it helps maximize our learning experience. It isn't science, that's for sure, as it's more of an art. But there is a method to it too. One important key to effective note taking is being able to write down enough notes for understanding the important points and ideas. If our notes are too few, it may not be enough for us to understand the important ideas and points come review time. Further, if we simply copy verbatim the instructor or presenter's bullet points, chances are high that we'll have a very hard time processing them later on during the review.

Take for example, these notes taken by an imaginary student in an imaginary class:

- Impt trig sol;
- Relvt acxsris; and
- Undertnd link.

Learning

Can you actually make sense of these notes? I don't think so, right? Right! On the other hand, notes are supposed to be just that – notes. We don't have to write everything down because doing so would keep us from understanding what the presenters discussing, particularly the important details. So we need to strike a balance – a sweet spot so to speak – in terms of writing to much or too little notes for effective learning. Here are some useful tips to do that:

- Write down key ideas, conclusions and central ideas;

- Note the presenter's statements preceded by emphasis statements such as "The point is", "In summary" or "More importantly", among others.

- Limit examples to just one and don't include in your notes digressions, off topic statements, jokes and stuff that you know you can easily research by yourself.

- Also note down sets of related ideas such as before-and-after, cause and effect and process steps.

- Annotate your notes using symbols for quicker notations such as asterisks (for important points), exclamation points (controversial or contestable points), + signs (multiple points working together) and arrows (time sequence or cause-and-effect relationships).

Learning

Chapter 16: Interleaved Practice

If you were to go about learning something new, memorizing new words or knowing how to solve an algebraic equation, how would you do it? For many, the plan of action would be to learn the basics, use related exercises for practicing, achieve a desire proficiency level then move on to the next topic for learning. This method is also known as block practicing, which is focusing on learning one thing or skill at a time. After repetitively practicing a newly learned skill for some time, we move on to another skill and basically repeat the whole thing.

This is where interleaved practice differs from block practicing. Interleaved practice involves learning or practicing more than one skill simultaneously on a parallel level.

Say there are 3 skill sets you want to learn – A, B and C. This is how a block practice session would visually appear:

AAA-BBB-CCC

On the other hand, here's how a session of interleaved practice would look like:

ABC-ABD-ABC (serial)

or

ACB-ABC-BCA (random)

The only "constraint" on the interleaved practice is that you can't work on the same problem combination consecutively or back-to-back.

Is It Effective?

Several studies pitting block and interleaved practices against each other have been done for evaluating both practices' effects. One of the latest studies on the two involved instructing students in the collegiate level on how to calculate the volumes of a wedge, spherical cone, half cone and spheroid. The students were classified into the Blockers – or the block practice people – and Mixers – the interleaved people.

The Mixers attended 4 tutorial sessions before doing 16 practice problems that were, well, mixed in such a way that each 4-problem set featured each of the volume problem types. On the other hand, the Blockers attended just one tutorial followed by solving 4 practice problems related to the tutorial subject before moving on to each of the 3 remaining volume problems in the same manner as the first.

The two groups both did 2 practices and an actual test – all spaced a week apart. The test results merely confirmed those of earlier studies on both practices – the Mixers scored 43% higher than the Blockers on the test.

How Does It Work?

Although there is no identified mechanism that precisely accounts for the efficacy of interleaved practice as a learning strategy, there are some theories that may help explain so. One is the Retrieval-Practice Hypothesis or RPH.

Our brains need to be able to access stored knowledge and transfer it to the working memory to be able to practice a particular skill. In block practicing, this happens only

Learning

during the start of the first practice problem and doesn't happen again during the other remaining practice problem solving sessions. During the interleaved practices, however, our brains are compelled to transfer the needed knowledge to the working memory during each and every practice problem solving session, which may result in the strengthening of neural pathways and increased knowledge retention.

To get a better idea of the RPH, picture yourself walking across a garden covered with Bermuda grass. Every time you walk across the lawn, you inevitably create a visibly broken in path on it. Think of block practice as walking to and fro only once while interleaved practice is walking to and fro several times on the lawn, which leaves a more distinguished path. The more you walk on the lawn, the more distinct and obvious the path becomes. In the same manner with interleaved practice, the more often you practice this way, the better a skill set is learned.

Another theory that may help explain the efficacy of interleaved practice is the Discriminative Contrast Hypothesis or DCH, which simply states that making our brains work simultaneously on learning multiple but similar skills compels it to differentiate between such skills. Another way of looking at it is that practicing just one skill repeatedly makes the brain expect the same in the future and thus, make it lazy in the sense that it doesn't work as hard at learning the other skills anymore. Because our brains are forced to distinguish the kind of skills needed for each problem set, it is compelled to focus harder, which may be the reason for the higher retention compared to the block practice.

Picture yourself driving your car down the freeway. When you set your car to cruise control and simply zone out, that's block practice. Stop and go traffic, on the other hand, is a good way to picture interleaved practice, which is a learning or practice strategy that keeps us more mentally engaged and on edge, which leads to better learning and retention.

Practical Tips For Using Interleaved Practice

The positive effects of interleaved practice have been documented in various studies, particularly in the areas of identifying birds, interpreting electrocardiograms, learning how to execute a badminton serve, differentiating painters' personal or artistic styles and learning simple motor skills. The various skills and knowledge and strong effects observed gives experts plenty of reason to believe that interleaved practice can be effective in terms of learning practically anything, if correctly utilized.

Some of the practical ways to incorporate interleaved practice in our daily learning activities include:

- Materials Study: It's important to first get instructions on that which we're trying to learn before we start practicing. We can't effectively practice if we have no clue on how to perform a certain skill or solve the problem.

- Practice With Purpose: For optimal learning, we shouldn't just practice for the sake of practicing. It should be with a clear goal in mind and the practice should work around towards achieving that goal.

- Against The Flow: The reason why block practice is inferior to interleaved practice in terms of learning is that it allows us to get into a groove – a flow so to speak. This makes us believe we already know the material we're trying to learn more than we actually do, which leads to complacency. Once it starts to become easy, shift to a different practice exercise – one that's more challenging or a break from the already established flow.

- Throw Some Old Stuff In: Remember the danger of getting into a flow or becoming familiar with the practice material? One good way to avoid falling into this trap is to throw in some older material or practice exercises that we've done before. It'll help keep things fresh and exciting, which is what interleaved practice does so well.

- Monitor Progress: One of the "dangers" of this technique is that it can be frustrating – even discouraging – even for the student who's very, very persistent. One way to minimize this risk of discouragement is to document the results of our practices to be able to see how we're actually progressing. This can effectively counter our perceived lack of progress, which can frustrate or discourage us.

Learning

Chapter 17: Self-Assessment

This learning technique involves regularly testing ourselves to determine how much of the study materials we are studying are we actually learning. It's beneficial in the sense that it helps us know if we really learned what we're supposed to learn or if we need to study more.

So how do we go about assessing ourselves? First, we'll need to collect the study materials that we'd like to test ourselves on. We can categorize these into 2 general ones: primary and processed. Primary materials include complete sources of information such as articles, audio recordings, books, glossaries, presentation slides and web pages. Processed materials include those that we made from primary ones that are more useful or truncated for us. These include idea maps, notes, outlines, paraphrases, study guides, and summaries.

Next, we test ourselves using both category of materials using different techniques like:

- Problem Flash Cards: With these cards, one side contains the problem to be solved and the answer or solution on the other. For example, one side may read "There are 2 bushels of apples with each bushel containing 100 apples. How many apples are there in all?" and the other will contain the answer.

- Question And Answer Cards: Instead of having two related terms – one on each side – these cards have questions on one side and the answers on the other.

- Vocabulary Flash Cards: These may contain 2 related terms with the main term on one side and the term that's related to or associated with the main term on the other side. Examples of these

Learning

combinations would be word and category, brand and generic names, word and meaning, sickness and cure and team and sport. It's important to remember with these kinds of flash cards is that they run both ways, i.e., backward and forward. What this means is we can start with either side of such cards for example, word and category or category and word.

- Close Test: This self-assessment technique takes a reading material you've already read and replaces every so number of words with blanks for you to fill up. After filling all the blanks, you check your answers for accuracy. For objectively maximizing the learning benefits of this technique, it's best if you do it with another person with the agreement that each of you will create close tests for the other. That way, the assessment questions and answers aren't biased.

- Create Matching Tests: Even if it sounds counterproductive – we'll always perfect them because we're the creator – it isn't. The learning value of this self-assessment technique doesn't lie in the test results but in the process of making the tests, where true learning happens.

- Matching Decks: Under this technique, we have many cards containing questions, answers and other related terms on the table. With all of them facing up, we'll try to pair all the related cards together, e.g., question and answer to the question, word and definition or problem and solution.

We can also make use of available prepared self-assessment materials found in most courses and textbooks that contain study materials or discussion questions designed for helping readers learn.

Learning

Lastly, we'll tally our scores and evaluate them accordingly. One way of maximizing the benefit of assessment is by doing it on a regular time interval, e.g., weekly, daily or monthly, in order for us to effectively monitor our progress or digress. Some helpful questions to ask to help us objectively assess our learning progress are:

- Did I miss anything?
- How did I score?
- Did I do better or worse than the previous assessments?
- Are my scores trending upward or downward and why?

To this extent, we'll also need to be able to monitor our progress through another learning technique called Self-Monitoring, which we'll discuss in the next chapter.

Chapter 18: Self-Monitoring

It's been shown in studies that paying attention to our learning progress helps improve our learning. Doing so makes it easier for us to remember and apply the new things we've learned as well as making it easy for us to develop skills. Although it may sound odd to say that we should pay attention to our learning, it shouldn't be. It simply means that we think about the things we have so far learned, the things we still need to learn and how well we are actually learning what we are trying to learn.

Primarily, we monitor our learning progress through sets of questions such as:

- How well do I understand the topic or material?
- Can I accurately summarize this topic or material?
- How can I rephrase this statement or idea?
- How well do I know the topic or material?
- What about the idea or material am I still unsure of?
- What are the things I still need to learn?
- Am I confident that I really know this topic or material?
- Do I know or remember the most important point of this material?

As much as its important to analyze what we did right, we also need to evaluate what we did wrong. I would agree with the thinking that between those who analyze their mistakes and those who analyze their correct answers, it is the former who actually learns something more significant.

Learning

Some questions to ask ourselves about our failures include:

- How come I didn't get this initially?
- What enabled me to finally get it?
- What led me to believe the wrong answer?
- Is there a consistent pattern to the questions I got wrong?
- How can I minimize these mistakes moving forward?

And speaking of asking questions, it's another technique we can use to accelerate our learning. Let's take a look at it in more detail, shall we?

Chapter 19: Asking Questions

It's been said that questions are signs of an active mind. I would agree with that. We can only ask relevant questions when we think about something. As such, it's also a good way to optimize our learning experiences.

Why? For one, asking questions help stimulate our curiosity, which is very important for learning and seeking answers. By simply asking questions, we become curious about the topic for learning even if initially, we weren't. This can prove to be very important when trying to learn very boring topics.

Asking questions also help us learn better by being able to clarify points and ideas that are unclear to us. Let's face it, some book and article authors and presenters try to be cool by being ambiguous or are simply not good at explaining things clearly. By asking presenters questions, e.g., examples, illustrations, clarifications, we get to clarify those that are not clear to us. It's quite different with authors and video presenters though. What we can do is to send them letters or emails to ask clarificatory questions for enlightenment. Worse comes to worse, we can just ask a friend or classmate who may have understood the point.

Asking questions also enable us to better understand by understanding the context in which points and ideas are presented. One of the best ways to learn something is by seeing the so-called "bigger picture" and by asking questions, we get to know the significance or role an idea or point that's unclear to us plays in the big picture and in doing so, we may be able clarify them.

Asking questions may seem pretty simple but for purposes of accelerating the learning experience, it's not as simple

Learning

as we think it is. Here are some ways we can ask questions for enhancing our learning experience:

- Journalist Approach: In every presentation or class, there are six journalistic questions that are usually answered or covered – Who, What, When, Where, Why and How. There are times, however, that some questions aren't covered and it's our responsibility – in the name of accelerated learning – to ask them.

- What's Next Approach: Asking "and then what?" is a very good way to encourage thinking forward or beyond the presentation and consider the unexplained or implicit ideas or consequences of those that were.

- Alternative Approach: Asking "what if?" or how the ideas or points presented would pan out if under a different set of circumstances helps us gain a much deeper understanding of ideas and points by showing us the extent of their validity.

Some very good general questions to ask include:

- What is the main point of the material or presentation?

- What evidences support the claims and conclusions made in the material or presentation?

- Is there any missing information?

- What is the presenter or author's point of view on the ideas and points presented and would this affect their validity?

Remember, asking questions help us learn better – and faster – by helping clarify important but ambiguous

Learning

points. The key is in the details and as such, it's worth keeping in mind that our questions should elicit the important and detailed answers we need to be able to fully understand and learn the ideas and points presented.

Chapter 20: Listen Actively

Today, we live in a high-stress, high-speed and high-tech society where communications has never been more important. The irony here is that as technology continues to improve, our ability to really "hear" each other may have even dwindled due to all the mental stimulation created by modern media.

That being said, good listening skills have become very rare these days. Such skills don't just help make us more accurate at work, minimize disagreements, enhance our understanding of others, address problems properly and strengthen relationships, it also helps us learn much, much better. Good listening skills, more than helping us listen, allows us to really hear what's being said.

Here are some practical ways to listen actively and develop great listening skills:

Eye Contact

Listening to someone talking while our head and eyes scan to and from the room can significantly affect our ability to really hear what people are trying to say or teach and as such, reduce our ability to learn well. It may also discourage or irritate the person who is talking to or teaching us that they'll just drop it and leave.

Eye contact is a given in most Western societies especially in terms of effective communications. When people talk, they establish eye contact. And of course, eye contact requires that the people talking are facing each other.

Facing the person talking and looking at their eyes is important for learning because this has the effect of

Learning

making us focus not just on their face but on everything they're trying to communicate through body language. Consider this experiment. Listen to a video podcast of say, Joel Osteen and then afterwards, watch the same podcast. Which among the two helped you learn his points better and kept you interested enough to focus? I bet it's the video podcast.

And that's why it's important for us to face the person and look at them in the eye for optimal learning.

Pay Relaxed Attention

After making eye contact, you must relax and avoid staring like a mad man or a stalker at the other person. Just look at them like you would during normal conversations. The main thing is that you're paying attention.

Part of the relaxed attention is screening out all forms of distraction such as noise and activity. Lastly, don't over-focus on the other person's mannerisms, accent or other characteristics that may become your distractions.

Open Your Mind

As you actively listen to the other person, remember to simply listen without mentally evaluating or judging what they say. If for some reason, what the other person said made you feel uncomfortable, it's alright to feel and acknowledge the feeling but don't let it escalate to the point that you're already judge because when that happens, effective listening for learning goes out the window.

It may be challenging at first to simply listen without reacting or concluding, especially to questionable statements. It'll help if we keep in mind that whatever the

Learning

other person says is merely a representation of their thoughts and feelings and not necessarily the truth or fact. Only by listening with an open mind can we truly hear what they're saying.

As kids, weren't we taught about how rude it is to interrupt someone in the middle of their sentence? It's a different generation these days where it's perfectly normal or even glorified to interrupt people in the middle of their sentences. So sad.

More than paying respects, cutting people off while in the middle of explaining something can also affect our ability to learn things well. Why? First, when we cut people off in the middle, we fail to hear the whole story and hence fail to learn the whole story. Second, cutting people off is a sign that we're so absorbed with our own version of the story that we brush off opportunities to learn better. What if at the end of their sentence comes the main point that points us to the error of our ways?

Picturesque Listening

Let yourself make a visual representation of the ideas or points that the other person is trying to communicate – be it a literal equivalent or a symbolic one. Remember, our brains think best in pictures and to the extent we can visualize what they're trying to say is the extent of our ability to learn what's being discussed well.

Don't Impose Opinion

Active listening also involves not imposing our opinions on others as if we're God and we know all truths perfectly. Apart from humility and courtesy, not imposing our opinions on anyone can indirectly help us learn much better from others. How? For one, we don't put ourselves in a position we're forced to save face when our opinions are eventually proven to be wrong. When we try to do that, we'll defend our positions – out of pride – even if it was wrong. We won't be able to learn and do the right thing because we're already in a position that we're compelled to protect our "integrity" and stand up for something that's already proven to be wrong just to save face.

When we don't impose but merely express when appropriate, we can learn from our mistakes graciously because we didn't impose and defended them as gospel truth. There's no shame because we acknowledge in the first place that those are opinions and so when they don't pan out, there's nothing to defend in the name of pride, which allows us to easily acknowledge the error of our ways and learn.

Wait Before Asking

Active listening also involves patience and timing. As such, part of it is waiting until the other person is done with what he or she is trying to say or has paused before asking questions. Not only is it courteous, it also gives the other person the opportunity to complete his or her statements and eventually satisfy our inquiry even before we ask.

Ask Relevant Questions Only For Clarifying And Understanding

And speaking of asking questions, we should ask relevant and clarifying questions only and avoid asking criticisms disguised as questions or off-tangent ones. Why? It's because asking irrelevant questions or criticisms disguised as such can cause the other person to veer off path and in the process, ruin his or her train of thought. This may cause them to present ideas and points in an irrelevant manner and thus, make it harder for us to learn what they're trying to impart.

Sadly, this happens to many people most of the time. Discussions and presentation going off tangent due to irrelevant questions or criticisms disguised as such. As the discussion sways off course, it's us the listeners who suffer the learning consequences.

Empathize

Putting ourselves in the other person's shoes helps us get a deeper and better understanding of the ideas and points they're presenting. I've had instances where I attended seminars where the speaker's background and point of reference were very close to my personal circumstances. When he explained it from that perspective, it was easy for me to grasp the concepts he discussed.

That's why empathy is important in active listening. When the heart and mind move in the same direction, learning is accelerated and optimized.

Feedback

Giving regular feedback to a speaker or presenter gives him or her the opportunity to learn how to present ideas better. At the end of the day, the real winners will be us – the audience or students. It's because – assuming they're open to feedback – they will adjust their presentation according to the feedback you gave in order to better drive home their points or expound on ideas, especially those that are quite complex. Giving them regular feedback is like giving them a target to aim for...bull's eye!

Hear What's Not Being Said

Active listening isn't just verbal listening – it also involves paying attention to non-verbal cues. It's been said that effective communications is just 10% verbal and the remaining 90% is non-verbal, i.e., body language.

A very good example, albeit a very unique one, is one of my favorite TV shows, Lie To Me. The show is about Cal Lightman – played by Tim Roth – who is a human lie detector contracted by the government to help catch crooks by determining if suspects are lying or not. He does this by reading facial expressions, body language and voice tone. There was an episode where in a suspected church bomber was being interrogated to find out where the next target is. Despite the suspect's reluctance to answer verbally, Lightman was able to learn from the suspect – just in the nick of time – the location of the next bombing target by merely reading the suspects body language.

In this case, you'll be able to know if the presenter is lying or isn't him or herself convinced of the truth of what they're presenting through their body language such as slouching, weak voice and inability to look at the audience.

You can also learn a lot about the people you care about – or want to care about – through non-verbal cues. For example, you're pitching your company's products to the purchasing manager of a department store. If you see the product manager yawning or not looking at you as you present, you learn that your presentation isn't doing well, which puts you in the position of being able to do it differently next time either with the same manager or other prospects.

Active Listening Workout

To help you hone your active listening skills, you can make use of another great learning technique – summarizing. Try to conclude your information-exchanging conversations with a summary sentence for 1 week at least. The point of this exercise is to make you aware of how actively you're listening – or not. If you know, you can make the necessary adjustments on your way to becoming an effectively active listener.

Learning

Chapter 21: Teach It To Learn It

Have you ever thought that you understand something very well only to have those dreams shattered when someone innocently asks you "why?" and you failed to answer that person satisfactorily? When asked to explain something you think you already understand well on a deeper level, do you experience a sensation of being stripped naked only to realize that afterwards the answer seems to have suddenly "materialized" in your mind?

If so, then you're like many other people who have experienced deeper learning of a topic as they sought to answer other people's questions or teach them about it. In fact, psychologists at the University of California at Berkeley found that explaining concepts verbally, especially to others, helps us understand them much better.

Why is that so? It's because deep inside, we have that intuitive ability to explain thoroughly, that's normally activated when explaining to another person. Other people's questions compel us to ditch our false sense of understanding of such concepts in favor of real reasoning.

According to Berkeley's Joseph Williams, we all have seemingly methodical intuitions as to what comprises a satisfactory explanation, which invokes an underlying principle. According to Williams, we want a reason or explanation that presents a broader pattern or framework and not merely specific to the issue at hand. As such, we are generally aware if the explanations given to us are satisfactory or not. On the other hand, we also have a general idea if we can explain something in the same terms when asked. It seems to be an intuitive characteristic for most of us, according to Williams.

Learning

That being said, Williams and his colleague Tania Lombrozo conducted a study in 2010 that showed people in general are able to better explain things when forced by others to do so. The bottom line? Explaining things to others helps us learn the underlying principle behind those things. This means we are able to learn much better. We're compelled to reassess what we think we know when other people ask us to explain.

Chapter 22: Other High Efficiency Study Methods

Are there more effective study methods a learner can adopt to make things easier? Any study method should benefit learners of different abilities, age groups, social backgrounds, or other settings. The methods should also help boost the academic performance based on various testing materials or conditions. In most cases, an effective study method doesn't demand for extensive learning in a bid to achieve the stipulated benefits.

Let's see some of the most effective study methods you can employ to make learning easier:

Practice Testing

As opposed to what its name suggests, this method doesn't demand that an actual test be done say in a specific testing environment. On the contrary, you can assess yourself any time, place and with any available testing material. For instance, you can test yourself with specific questions and comparing your replies to the correct answers. Alternatively, you can use flash cards or attend other tests in different testing environments.

Practice testing mainly works due to two main reasons:

1. Testing can facilitate the encoding of other effective mediators through targets and cues. Current research found out that practice testing could boost the ability to mentally organize your knowledge thus increase the speed and extent of information to be retrieved.

2. Testing can enhance retention of content as it triggers elaborative retrieval processes as you gauge your long-term memory and retrieve associated information.

Practice testing is recommended as it addresses the time demand factor, since it doesn't require long durations to learn how to do things. The method can also work for various types of subjects or tasks. That said, there is evidence that immediate retesting without allowing 'reasonable' time between tests doesn't boost learning process. Thus you should aim to only assess yourself after a specific time frame has elapsed and when ready to do tests.

Distributed Practice

In this study method, you simply divide your studies over specific time intervals as opposed to having to do one large chunk. Based on distributed practice, you don't have to cram tests! Adopting this study method can help you learn as your brain has enough time to store information as it switches back and forth through the focused and diffused mode of thinking. When you space your studies, research shows that the brain has an easier time retrieving what you've already learnt.

A specific 1979 research revealed that learners who distributed their study sessions with a set interval of 30 days between each session were the best performers in tests done 30 days after last study session. The findings also showed that students who distributed their sessions with only a day between each session performed slightly worse than the first group. In the same research, learners who didn't allow any time between sessions were the worst performers, and actually achieved terrible results compared to the two groups.

Most learners wouldn't manage a 30 days luxury in academic sessions bearing in mind that semesters only take 3-4 months in length. Most courses also feature 2-4 big tests in between the semesters alongside weekly tests and homework. Thus, the best way to use distributed learning is to adopt a 24-hour spacing interval before you restudy the material. After attending the first few days of study, try to space out the forthcoming classes between 24 hours spacing.

Once you have reviewed your first 4 sessions within a 24 hours spacing between each review, you can further space them out without much details. In some cases, you may allow a month to elapse after the first 4 review sessions before you proceed. To further boost your learning speed, try to combine the practice testing with distributed practice. Research has shown that learners who are able to merge both study methods can achieve high marks in exams.

Elaborative Interrogation

This can be defined as the process where you answer the question "WHY" in a bid to grasp information or understand concepts. For example, if you are studying about $E=MC^2$, you can try to find out why does E equals the said MC^2? Elaborative interrogation can be easy to adopt but may demand that you understand the said topic fully. With time, you can efficiently use this interrogation to study as research shows that you need 4 more minutes to understand concepts through this method compared to a reading-only approach. Good news is that reading can be monotonous for some learners and thus elaborative interrogation can be done alongside reading in a bid to make learning fun.

However, the method can be limited in its application as might only fit to answer factual statements such as $E=MC^2$. Thus, try to frequently use the method throughout your reading and pause to ask yourself questions within each paragraph or sub-topic. You can also get a notebook to write down the quizzes that get to your mind alongside possible answers to them. The questions and answers can help to further expand your long-term memory.

Highlighting

This method comprises of highlighting, underlining as well as other methods to mark study materials. Highlighting can be recommendable because it's easy to practice and apply, as it requires a little or no training. However, research shows that learners who use highlighting as a study method may not achieve noticeable improvement in their scores. The reason for this is that highlighting can only be effective or applicable only to limited tasks or information, and may need to be paired with other methods to work.

That said, you can pair highlighting with other effective study methods in order to boost your ability to retain information. For example, try methods such as self-testing or recall in order to further internalize information learned or highlighted.

Rereading

This concept is based on the theory that reading can boost learning effectiveness as it increases the total amount of details encoded not considering the level or kind of information that a study material contains. On the other head, the technique doesn't require any special training. Though majority of learners prefer to re-read content in a bid to permanently retain information, you may not get much out of the time you invest to re-read. To some learners, the concept can be viewed as a diminishing return on investment as one might only gain little or no new information after the first rereading.

For learners who prefer to read content multiple times, try to skip just a little time before the next re-reading session. Research shows that learners who allow an interval of 4 days between the initial reading and the re-reading session can actually improve their performance. In between the spacing you choose, just move ahead to other topics and then repeat the first content read after about 4 days. In so doing, you both read new information as you remember the old information every day.

Think-Pair-Share

About 5 minutes of class time can do wonders in terms of content learnt! In this study method, a tutor can hand out pencils and index cards and then set a 90 seconds timer for students to raise points about a chosen topic. Once a timer sounds, a teacher can ask students to work in pairs for another 90 seconds in a specific and ritualized manner. The main objective is to come up with those ideas they share in common with members of the group within the 90 seconds. The answers or ideas may be a synthesis of their previous comments, and should be an agreed upon idea that they share.

Before learners get to work in groups, each member should read their initial ideas or answers while others listen. Research shows that when learners are given a chance to be heard while reading can motivate them to be responsible of their own learning. The think-pair share concept work in the view that writing down content and then reading to other person can assist introverts to express themselves without having to speak before a group. The concept also helps students to feel equal and respected even when holding different opinions on affairs. The last 90 seconds should be used by learners in a group to read their contribution and come up with common ideas.

Question Stacking

This is another method to reinforce equity in classes or in departmental meetings. An organiser of a meeting or class can ensure that when someone is about to make a comment their name is first written down a paper. Then you go through the paper and request for comments. Ensure that no other person should make a second comment or ask another question until every other learner on the sheet has gone first. It's also recommended to set a time limit of say 30-60 seconds per question, as the respondents get used to the timings. This learning method helps set a practice of respect, responsibility and consideration in a ritualized manner.

The Exit Ticket

The method is basically for tutors or leaders in learning environments. Ensure that you end each class 3 minutes before time, say through the assistance of a timer. Then provide index cards for students to write a question by the end of the lesson, in full sentence and signed. You can also open a Google Doc to be shared with other learners both in the institution and globally. Each of the learners should write down a well-structured question that should form the kind of post-class introspection. Tutors can use these questions to help develop respective lessons, and the index card can help you take roll call on attendance and make learning fun.

Active Learning

Active learning is a method that is meant to boost learning or teaching in various classes. This learning method demands for a deeper planning on top of just leading learners through ordinary classroom. Learning is termed as active if it can change the sense of long-term memory. Simply put, the term applies to any kind of learning engaged by students in a class as opposed to just passively listening to the teacher. When a learner is fully engaged in learning, one can easily decide their level of learning activity; say through note taking or other thoughtful consideration.

Proponents of this concept state that for active learning to take place, it should take place within the student's brain as opposed to the observed behavior that is a means to that cognitive work.

A teacher should guide the learner in active learning, and trigger those cognitive events in rhythm with the expected learning outcomes. The classroom activities normally have defined objective and should guide you toward your desired learning goals. There are about 5 techniques that can be used to make active learning both fun and effective; i.e. structured sharing; team quizzes, students acting as teachers, using listening teams and just-in-time teaching. Let's briefly see how you can learn through these methods:

Just-in-time Teaching

As a learner, you simply need to complete an assessment or assignment on any topic before the class period, and then have your instructor review your work. The tutor should in the process adapt discussions or activities based on the common errors, misconceptions, or problems that you have concerning a topic. The instructor may use course management system say like a blackboard or a web-based assessment package.

Listening Teams

Here you can create groups of four learners with each of you having a different role to play. If you have an instructor, you can mix up roles within classes or between classes in a bid to fully engage all learners. The learning teams should facilitate learners and offer a chance for discussion or questions on key course concepts. For example, let's see how 4 learners can form a listening team on their own even without facilitation of an instructor:

- ✓ Learner 1: To highlight applications or examples of key concepts
- ✓ Learner 2: Come up with three clarifying questions about the concept.
- ✓ Learner 3: Evaluate which areas of the topic causes misconceptions and try to explain why
- ✓ Leaner 4: Point 2 or 3 areas of agreement with textbook material and explain why it's so.

Your material for study can be anything ranging from a textbook, video tape or actual lecture. Listen or read the material and then come up with areas where there's a misconception or questions. You can then constitute a 5-10 minutes meeting to share ideas and to agree on key points. The groups can share concepts and ask questions from fellow groups or the lecturer to get better understanding.

Learning

Structured Sharing

This technique should help you review the content of a class project or presentation from multiple points of views. In reviewing your content, you can assess whether you have learnt anything new and come up with relevant questions on the topic. A class of 20-30 learners can work well where each student has three 3" x 5" cards to raise ideas. Within 15-20 minutes, an instructor or group leader can come up a superlative to be addressed. Ideas to be focused on include the most confusing topic, most trivial, difficult or those quite amusing. Follow these steps:

-Let the group leader or instructor pass three blank 3" x 5" cards to each group member.

-Each member should at the end of the session write down 3 main things you have chosen to be addressed; E.g. three most difficult words to pronounce.

-At the end of the session, the leader or instructor should collect the cards from each group member alongside his or her ideas.

-Before the next class, have the cards reviewed in order for your understanding of the topic to be assessed. A lecturer or other expert can help assess how students' responses matched with the intended content. From here, an instructor can decide area to be clarified and where to elaborate further.

-The group leader or instructor should then instruct members to reveal their replies alongside those of their peers.

-Come the next session, an instructor can give each member 3-4 of the cards including theirs until all cards have been shared.

Learning

-Each member should select a card that they most concur with. Each member should be allocated 30-60 seconds to explain why he or she picked a certain card and his or her reasons behind that decision.

-Each member should review those cards and understand how others thought about the same topic, in a bid to learn something new and frame their learning accordingly.

Students as the Teachers

In this learning technique, you need to prepare a real lesson to a certain topic preferably that's your choice. Your lesson can be about 10 minutes long meant for a smaller group of students or a 30-40 minute long session for the entire class. As opposed to an ordinary or simple class presentation that most learners may have been used to, here you must prepare a lesson in the most professional manner.

Ensure that you include learning outcomes commonly known as lesson objectives, the discussion questions, a form of practice, and another form of evaluation! You should also encourage your 'class' to ask you questions and address those misconceptions that your audience may have about the topic. If you may want to use this technique to evaluate your learning skills, the first thing to do is create a basic lesson outline for your learners to follow. These tips can come in handy:

-Try to explain basic teaching skills to your 'class'

-State how you will assess the performance of your students on tasks that you assign them. For instance, you can assess them based on how they adhere to the lesson outline or based on their peers' performance on the same topic

Learning

-You can have an instructor supervise the lesson or alternatively request for teacher evaluation sheets to assess your class

-Ensure that you create clear-cut topics that your students may enjoy and understand

-Provide examples of credible resources for the lesson preparation and future reference

-Let your students illustrate their creativity as well. For instance, you can pair them into pairs and let them work out tasks as a team.

At the end of the lesson, ensure a more experienced person can assess you as well. A supervisor can help assess your performance on lesson preparation and delivery. Your score can be based on your preparedness, ability to cover the topic, presentation method and your ability to evaluate your "students".

Research has shown that having a student act, as a teacher is an effective way to make them active in their learning process. For students to effectively prepare and deliver their lessons, they ought to first develop interest and understand the topic well. Thus, they can develop deeper insight and will have ownership of their selected topic.

Team Quizzes

This technique can help to review learners based on understanding the topic as well as exam preparation if done in a careful manner. Learners should be divided in three teams; where team 1 attempts to answer short quiz while team 2 and 3 review their notes. A few rules can help make team quizzes effective:

Learning

-One team should be assigned the role to create a certain set of questions, based on the outline and other course materials.

-The other 2 teams should study the outline and the materials collectively.

-Groups should have sufficient time to study the materials and prepare the questions.

-Once groups are well constructed and fully prepared, the first group presents the questions they have to the members of the two groups.

-If team 2 misses a quiz, the 3rd team should be given the chance to answer. The next quiz should go to team 3 and then the missed questions should be reverted to team 2.

-If team quizzes is to repeated for another round, different set of students should get the chance to create the questions.

Chapter 23: Lifestyle

"Your genetics load the gun. Your lifestyle pulls the trigger." – Dr. Mehmet Oz, celebrity doctor.

One thing young people often take for granted is lifestyle. Well, at least I know I did. Back in the day, I could party practically the whole night, sleep for just 2 hours and work out at the gym the next day before going to the office. These days, I'm like those zombies in the Walking Dead in front of my office computer on days where I don't sleep enough the night prior. It is at my age when reality starts to kick in. For me in particular, it started on my 3rd decade.

It may be that genetically, we are blessed with mutant-like mental powers but the way we live our lives will eventually determine if we'll be able to fully exercise those powers or not. Our I.Q. may be the same level as that of Albert Einstein but what good would that be if we're too high or sleepy on most of our waking hours? Worse, what good would such mutant mental powers be to a corpse?

We may have the power but our lifestyles hold the key to unleashing it.

Stress

Stress is one of those factors that have a great impact on our ability to learn things, both positive and negative. Generally speaking, there are 2 kinds of stress based on their effects on the human body. Eustress and distress. Eustress is considered the good kind of stress, which can be a catalyst for physical and personal growth. Distress, on the other hand, is the "villain" stress, which can propel us into sicknesses, decreased ability to learn and other negatively sorry states of existence.

Learning

One good example of the good stress is that which we experience when we lift weights to build strength and muscles. As we lift barbells or dumbbells, we put stress on our muscles, which at the right amounts, causes muscular and physical strength growth.

On the other hand, applying the same kind of stress but at levels that are considered excessively dangerous for our current strength and conditioning levels, can lead to injuries like torn muscles or worse, broken bones. In the gym I used to work out in, I know of someone who practically tore his thumb off as the barbell he was lifting during a squat exercise fell on said body part after he fainted from overexertion.

When it comes to mental distress, there are several causes for such. One is **clutter**. Based on a Princeton University Neuroscience Institute's study that was featured in the Journal of Neuroscience, the presence of many visual stimuli (as in the case of clutter) compete for neural representation, the result of which is one chaotic mental environment that impedes our ability to focus and process information and consequently, to maximize learning.

We can look at clutter as a toddler demanding your attention while you're rushing a report that your company's Board of Directors wants to be submitted in 30 minutes – it impedes optimal focus and learning.

Between the 2 kinds of clutter – mental and physical – the latter is usually easier to clear. And the best way to do it is by organizing our things. But if like me, you find keeping your stuff organized as easy as manually solving an astrophysics equation, it may be in your best interests to read materials on how to successfully do so. It seems that there is a method to the madness that is clutter management and books such as Go Organize by Marily Bohn and The One-Minute Organizer by Donna Smallin make for great resources that can greatly assist such an ambitious mission.

Procrastination – or rest now, do later – is another great source of mental distress that can seriously affect our ability to maximize learning. I was once a chronic procrastinator and believe me it can be so stressful. I would always put off working out at the gym because often times, I feel "tired" after office hours. I figured it's best to work out when my energy levels are at an all time high. But because such an energy level is at best, as common as a blood moon, I never really got around to doing it until I've already gained so much weight and I only had a couple of weeks before summer starts and I'll have to hit the beach and bare me body! I had to cram all that fat-burning training in a few short weeks via severe calorie restriction and super-intense workouts. The result? Strained relationships and significantly reduced work performance. Lesson? Do what you can now while there's still time and don't put off what can be done today for tomorrow if you don't want your stress levels to go haywire.

Finally, mental distress can also come from **taking on excess commitments, obligations or responsibilities**. We have to admit that we're only human and as such, we are limited in our ability to mentally process stuff. There will be moments when the mere thought of more duties and responsibilities to fulfill the ones we're currently working on will be enough to tire and burn us out mentally, which can significantly affect our ability to maximize learning. The only way to minimize the risk of this happening is to set clear personal boundaries as to how much responsibilities, obligations and commitments we should take at any given time. For this purpose, calendars and planners can be of great help to us, which allows us to see the bigger picture of our personal schedules that can help us stave off the temptation or tendency to take on too much on our plates.

Learning

And when we're not mentally overwhelmed, our ability to learn is maximized.

Oh, I'm sorry – I focused so much on bad stress that I haven't discussed good mental stress yet. Without good stress, a.k.a., eustress, our mental capacities won't grow as our muscles do. In fact, our mental performance may even atrophy (shrink) without eustress.

Why is this so? It's because just as with lifting weights or running long distances, our mental abilities – including capacity to learn new things – grow as we continue to gradually increase the mental workload we take on. By regularly subjecting our minds to moderately good levels of stress, we expand its capacity to perform, including learning.

One of the best ways to positively stress our minds is reading. Personally, I find this to be a very good way to learn a lot of new things, which is particularly important in my line of work. Consider this e-book you're reading now. This is a product of years of reading many books on different topics, which expanded my mind's ability to learn new things and consequently, write this book.

Mental exercises and games are 2 more great sources of mental eustress. When we always subject our minds to challenges, it adapts to them much like our physical muscles adapt to increasing workloads, resulting in a more powerful and efficient mind. An excellent way to exercise our minds is by playing puzzles like Sudoku or crosswords and strategy games such as games of the generals, chess and checkers, among others.

If not sure of where to begin from, you can try these simple steps:

Learning

✓ Pick a new sport

Some sports require both brain and body coordination, and stress application on the brain cells helps them grow. The more complicated the activities the better. This is because the brain takes these new activities as challenges, which can help to improve your memory.

✓ Have a walk

Taking a short leisurely walk in the morning can help your brain to grow. When you do this, make sure to incorporate the atmosphere around you, taking everything that is happening into context. Try to analyze the smells you come across, the sounds and music, and everything that is happening. This helps to keep your mind alert throughout the day and prevents it from slipping into boredom.

✓ Do cardio

For effective mental performance, take a short time to do some simple sweaty exercises such as jumping a rope, a sprint run, or squat bend. You can do these quick exercises before going into an exam room, a conference briefing, or giving a speech.

Once accustomed to light exercises, increase intensity to realize better results. Take vigorous and moderate exercises that may amount to a loss of about 350 calories thrice weekly. You can do this by enrolling to a local gym or subscribing to an online training manual that will guide you through the exercises.

Learning

✓ Learn new vocabularies

To improve your thinking and word skills, try reading as much as you can and learn a new vocabulary every day. Reading magazines and books can be a great way to exercise your brain. You can also learn a new language. This exercise trains the part of your brain that stores language and can even help you speak your own language better.

✓ Challenge yourself

Challenges such as learning to use your other hand or learning to play a musical instrument can help you exercise your brain. Using your left hand helps to exercise the left side of your brain while playing musical instruments helps you to tune your brain finely while keeping it in shape at the same time.

✓ Get in a team

Socializing with people by talking about matters such as politics, religion or any challenging discussions makes your brain grow healthy. Make learning continuous by going back to school, or taking free lessons if you don't have money. There are lots of free lessons available online that you can make use of to help work out your brain. You can also train your brain by learning a new skill like dancing, music, or arts. These help to train different parts of your brain. You can also join a group with people you share similar interests such as a hobby, career or responsibility.

Try yoga exercises

Doing yoga can help you focus for longer and also boost your blood circulation, cardio health and lower stress levels. Yoga is particularly effective when done for 10-15 minutes daily through a series of body movements. Even if you feel moody and tired, yoga can instantly boost your concentration, clear your mind and relax the body. Look for a yoga instructor or try beginner yoga poses at your house for no added cost. Try the following yoga techniques:

Squat

Keep the feet slightly apart, as you stand with raised hands to shoulder level.

-Then push the knees together to appear as if you are seated onto an imaginary chair. Bend the knees as far as you can. Squats help tone muscles of the thighs and glutes, and can make you get more balance and control for your body.

Plank pose

Planking can strengthen your cores and boost your balance to ensure you appear younger and healthy.

-Start by getting down with your hands and knees, and then balance the toes as you raise the body up.

-Ensure that the entire body is in a single line, starting from the feet to head. Also maintain the arms straight with the palms flat on the ground.

Seated twist

-Be seated cross-legged on the ground, and then hold the right knee using the left hand.

-Then stretch the right hand outward in order to have the palm touch the floor behind the back. Now twist the torso in order to look back.

Learning

This pose should twist your stomach muscles and tone these muscles, and can also reduce double chin and boost your flexibility

Downward dog pose

This pose is very effective at boosting your flexibility, circulation and strengthening the spine.

-Get to all fours with the hands and on the feet placed flat on the ground. Maintain the feet hip width apart.

-Then raise the hips in order the body to create a V shape, and pull the belly button close to the spice. Allow the hand to hang.

Warrior pose

- Feet apart, stand straight with the left foot pointing outwards. Keep the torso straight and the right foot inward. Now exhale and bend the left knee; and inhale as you stretch the arms out.

-Then turn the head to look at your left arm and hold the pose for around 10 seconds. Repeat the pose on the other side.

Alternatively, you can try the pose by keeping the right arm on the right knee instead of stretching the arms parallel to the floor. Then raise the left arm over the head. You should look up to see the tip of the right hand.

Tree pose

Do the pose from a standing pose with both feet next to each other and your arms placed on the side.

-Position the left sole onto the right calf and then fold the hand together. Hold against the chest or above the head. Then hold this pose for around 10 seconds and repeat.

Sphinx pose

The pose is very suitable in making the chest and spine healthy as well as toning the upper arms. While lying face down, tuck the elbows on the sides.

-Inhale and put some pressure on your palms in order to lift the head and chest. Maintain the elbows on the ground and hold this pose for about 5 inhales or exhales.

Forward bend pose

The exercises are effective at warming you up, toning the joints and hips, and boosting the blood circulation to the head. It should help you remain fit, younger, and supple.

-Begin with palm on the ground, inhale, and then lift the hands up. Then bend forward as you exhale and touch the palm onto the ground.

-Hold your breath and inhale as you rise up, and repeat the exercise about 10 times.

Doing physical and mental exercises is important for a few reasons. First, regular exercise raises the level of oxygen supplied to the brain, thus improving the level of concentration and ability to retain and incorporate information into your memory. Apart from this, regular exercise helps to break down calories that may cause illnesses such as diabetes and some cardiovascular diseases, which may cause memory loss. Furthermore, when you exercise, you enhance the functionality of brain chemicals and help protect your brain cells.

For more ways to train the mind, check out the website www.lumosity.com, which is where scientists study neuropsychological activities and design new ones in the form of challengingly fun mental activities and games. In the true sense of the word, it's a good way and fun way to stress our minds for optimal performance.

Sleep

It can't be disputed – inadequate sleep means poor mental performance. It's because as with all other muscles in the body, our brains also need adequate time to recharge, rest and recuperate. With enough rest (via sleep), we stay focused, alert, awake and quick to respond. Otherwise, we have difficulty focusing, staying alert, keeping awake and responding promptly – classic symptoms of strained mental performance.

Just how much sleep do we really need for optimal learning? Unfortunately, there's no real objective, one-size-fits-all benchmark for that. However, it's an acceptable estimate that on average, we need anywhere between 7 to 10 hours of sleep for peak mental performance, including learning new stuff, depending on a person's lifestyle.

To get a more personalized estimate of your sleep requirements, try waking up without an alarm for a couple days straight. Write down how many hours you slept every day before waking up on your own and how you felt during the day. With this simple activity, you can get a good estimate of your optimal sleeping requirement for accelerated learning and overall peak mental performance.

Sleep plays a critical role in memory because consolidation of new information learnt takes place when you are asleep. Good sleep before learning a new thing makes the mind fresh to accommodate new information. Studying when you are sleep deprived limits your level of concentration and you cannot learn much. Let's see other ways to help you sleep better:

- Gauge how much sleep you get in one day. You can do this by calculating the number of hours you sleep at night by recording your sleeping time, waking time and the length of time you woke up at night.

- Stop watching late night T.V. If you are an early riser, you should consider the time you go to sleep and decide if watching late night shows affects your sleeping time. Some programmes can be addictive and it is advisable to refrain from watching them at all.

- If you are a fun of video games, limit the time you take playing them at night. However, some video games could be tactical and challenging in a manner to help improve your brain cells, don't get carried away. Make time for them and allocate sufficient naptime so that you get enough sleep.

- During the day say on a hot day, take a nap to help your brain reflect on the day's activities and relax. A nap could help recover some of the sleep you may have lost during the night.

- Avoid any hobbies that may be keeping you from enjoying a good night's sleep. Consider cutting it of or rescheduling your timetable to accommodate hobbies that cannot be skipped. No matter how fun it may be, if it is keeping you late at night, it is not healthy for you.

Socials

It's reported by an organization called AARP or the American Association of Retired Persons that a study of 116,000 people, those who were considered to have strong relationships experienced less mental performance decline than those who didn't have such relationships. Other experts have also opined that deterioration of mental performance can be accelerated by social isolation. Possible reasons for this include being deprived of opportunities to be excited, to learn and experiencing fun and surprise – all of which are important for optimal mental performance. And that includes learning. Www.fitbrain.com also reports that opportunities to socialize combined with our individual talents can optimize our brain's health.

If socializing was not your thing, you can adopt a few self-improvement steps to ensure you satisfy your emotional needs. You need to determine if your need for each of the following is met:

✓ Need for friendship

The initial step is to be around other people in order to make new friends. It does not have to be with the popular crew, but being able to make a real friend can prove useful when you are in need. You can also join an organization, group or club with people you share similar interests. You can take advantage of social websites such as Twitter or Facebook to meet new people. Joining a team, such as a sport team, band, or choir with a laid back attitude, without a competitive mindset, can also be a great way to make friends with people in the team.

✓ Need for respect

If you are looking to get respect, you need to first respect others. Try not to badmouth other people, and if there is a problem, try addressing the issue first hand instead of talking behind their back. On the other hand, you need to also respect yourself by taking care of your appearance, and standing up for yourself. Research shows that being

Learning

loved and respected can boost your confidence, and likewise help you socialize and learn new stuffs.

✓ Need for affection

Everyone needs affection thus you should find a good friend, or participate in any available free hugs campaign around you. You don't have to go overboard to get affection. Even holding hands and having a nap on your partner's lap can be relaxing and comforting. You can also create your own if you are outgoing enough. In addition, you can also join an online community that you feel comfortable about and make friends.

✓ Need for serving others

Being of service to others in need can be a source of joy for you and those you are helping. It does not have to be much. You can even volunteer at hospitals, social service agencies or shelters by offering your services to those in need. These activities are offer a nice chance to get educated on other fields that you cannot cover during ordinary coursework.

Whatever you do to socialize, ensure that you surround yourself with positive, supportive, and encouraging people! This is because being around negative people no-doubt has a negative effect on you. The first thing to do is evaluate those around you i.e. the people in your life. Seek out team members, friendships, relationships, and even companions with people who can add value to your life and facilitate learning.

So if you want to experience optimal learning and mental performance, have fun! Go out and socialize!

Chapter 24: How to Eat To Boost Your Memory and Learning

Memory and the learning process is basically affected by your mind and the ability to process information. But now and then the brain can get fatigue after a challenging task or assignment, right? Research has shown that taking the right foods can help boost your memory and learning process. A proper diet can help stimulate release of "feel good" brain chemicals namely tryptophan and serotonin. These brain chemicals control how you feel and your ability to absorb information.

You need to consume a balanced diet to ensure that the brain is performing optimally without breakdown. To start you off, try to get these top 30memory enhancing foods:

1. Dark Chocolate

Dark chocolate is one snack you should never forget to pack in your bag, especially for a cocoa chocolate with a 70 percent cocoa or higher! This is because research has shown that cocoa has an active ingredient that helps boost the serotonin levels in the brain. Eaten in moderate amounts, Chocolate can help boost the level of serotonin in the brain. Cocoa is also rich in polypherols and anti-oxidants and can help to boost sensitivity to insulin.

The best type is the pure dark chocolate, which doesn't contain added ingredients, and can as well reduce your brain's stress levels. Chocolate is able to reduce cortisol level, the hormone that causes stress and anxiety. Ensure that you don't end up consuming excess amounts as chocolate may cause problems with your metabolism. Chocolate can have high amount of sugars and may spike your blood sugar level, which reduces effectiveness of serotonin.

2. Wheat germ

A germ is the part of a plant that develops into a new species, also referred to as the embryo. Wheat germ is the most nutritious part of the wheat kernel, as it has high concentration of choline. This chemical is what your body requires to manufacture acetylcholine, a memory-enhancing neurotransmitter. You need about 550 milligrams of choline in a day, whereas 100 grams of wheat germs can offer about 152 milligrams of choline. Wheat germ is one of the foods that has ample amount of memory-enhancing chemicals.

3. Blueberries

Many people may not appreciate the blue color of the fruit but blueberries can be a healthy food choice for you. This fruit is rich in anti-oxidants, substances that help combat free radicals, environmental toxins that enters the body and damages the body cells. A study done by Tufts University reveals that polyphenols can help reduce the rate of inflammation and also offer better communication in neurons. This facilitates the brain to perform optimally and process required information within a shorter duration. On the other hand, antioxidants in this fruit can help create cognitive pathways in the brain to reduce effects of poor memory as you age.

4. Avocados

Avocados are the healthiest fruits you should consume regularly due to the mono-unsaturated fats it contains and omega 3 fatty acids. The good fats in avocado do not cause cardiovascular diseases and instead help to control blood sugar levels and restore a smooth shiny skin. Avocados are healthy to the brain due to the folate and vitamin K that helps to prevent blood clots in the brain, which work to prevent stroke. Folate helps to improve memory, concentration, and cognitive function. In a study to demonstrate effectiveness of avocadoes, people who eat avocadoes regularly were found to have a lower risk of developing Alzheimer's disease by about 67 percent.

On the other hand, avocadoes have a high quality protein and low sugar content compared to other fruits. You also get vitamin B and C, both of which your body doesn't store and which need to be replenished daily. You need to eat about ¼ cup of avocado daily to get required nutrients. Try adding avocadoes to your smoothies, salads, side dishes, or dips and also eat as snack to replace the bad fats in baked products.

5. Bananas

Research has shown that eating bananas after training can help restore the electrolytes lost and improve brain functionality. Banana is rich in carbohydrates and tryptophan, which helps boost serotonin production. Banana is also rich in magnesium, a mineral that helps in excretion of ammonia from the body to prevent interruption of brain functions. Once proteins are digested, the body generates ammonia, which can disrupt cognitive function even in smallest amounts.

Your body requires about 265 to 350 milligrams of magnesium mineral daily to facilitate electrical functions that happen in brain cells. A large banana should provide you with about 37 milligrams of magnesium. Though bananas are rich in sugar and are of high glycemic index, you can eat them in moderation to boost your mental function. Aim to eat few bananas for breakfast, mix with whey protein to prepare a shake or eat as post-training snack. Also, try to simmer half a banana in coconut milk for a dessert to strengthen the brain after a hard task and to improve sleep.

6. Spinach

Dark leafy greens are recommended due to their potential to enhance brain function and inhibit possible oxidative stress. Spinach has a high amount of magnesium, a mineral that neurons rely on to send messages in the brain. Magnesium can help inhibit the over-activation of nerve receptors, which is caused by other neurotransmitters like glutamate. Lack of magnesium can allow glutamate to over-activate the receptors and cause cellular damage and decrease in cognitive response. Eating 3 servings of spinach daily can help combat cognitive decline by a whopping 40 percent!

7. Peanut Butter

Nutritional experts recommended that you eat healthy fats from foods like peanut butter, avocado, coconut oil and wild caught fatty fish. Peanut butter has around 8 grams of protein in every 2 tablespoons you consume. Further studies show that it has folate, a mineral that helps boost memory function as well as the brain's processing speed. The B-vitamins in peanut butter can help control proper brain function while vitamin E can protect your brain from damage caused by chemical breakdown. Other minerals like potassium, phosphorus, copper, and magnesium facilitate the nerve cells to produce electrical signals in a bid to enhance communication.

8. Eggs

Eggs are a source of protein, omega 3 fatty acids and other nutrients required by your body. This protein food is rich in choline, a B vitamin that helps fight defects like dementia while boosting memory and mental awareness. Eggs can boost your serotonin levels since they contain high quality omega 3 fatty acids among them the long chain D.H.A and E.P.A. These fats have been known to improve both the mood and the serotonin levels in the brain. On the other hand, eggs are rich in cholesterol, which has shown to boost testosterone hormone and serotonin levels.

Though cholesterol is linked to cardiovascular diseases, a couple of studies have shown that lower cholesterol level causes brain drain, depression and mood swings. A recent research has shown that unhealthy brain and total cholesterol levels were inversely related. Having a high amount of testosterone can also help boost muscle gain and fat loss.

9. Broccoli

This veggie is rich in choline and vitamin K, nutrients that help boost memory and cognitive function. Broccoli also provides vitamin C and fiber, which ensure you remain fuller for longer without the disturbing cravings. A serving of broccoli should provide you with about over 2,000 micrograms of vitamin K that is known to boost brainpower. The veggie can match with a number of recipes such as soups, smoothies, pesto dips and as snack.

A study done in London showed that broccoli is vital in treatment of Alzheimer's disease due to a presence of chemical called glucosinolates. Another chemical called sulforaphane has shown to reduce risk of brain damage that can develop from other related injuries. Dieters who regularly eat broccoli are often sharper than those who don't eat the veggie due to these chemical compounds.

10. Buckwheat

This natural starch contains high amount of B vitamins and tryptophan compared to other sources of starchy carbs. The B vitamins are vital for addressing mental fatigue, depression and boosting energy levels. Vitamin B6 for instance helps maintain a regular production of serotonin in the brain. Based on various studies, you need to include at least one source of starchy carbs that increase serotonin levels in order to boost memory and learning process.

This carb also contains dchiroinositol, an anti-diabetic nutrient that can suppress high blood sugar levels. Natural sources of starch work by causing a little insulin spike to help eliminate other amino acids from the bloodstream, and tryptophan enters the blood and is eventually processed into serotonin. Though starchy foods can boost the synthesis of serotonin, you'll also need protein tryptophan which acts as a fuel in production of serotonin. Ensure that you consume moderate level of carbs in order to balance insulin as well as serotonin levels. Eat more carbs later in the day together with other serotonin boosting foods for better results.

11. Almonds

Nuts have high antioxidant content which fights free radicals responsible for brain damage and are also loaded with vitamin E. This vitamin can help improve Alzheimer's symptoms and boost mental alertness. Almonds have high content of zinc, a mineral that is used to balance mood. An almond has healthy fats and iron, a nutrient that inhibit brain fatigue. Such problems in the brain lead to mood disorders and brain failure.

On the other hand, almonds provide riboflavin, L-carnitine and phenylalanine which have shown to feed the brain. These substances also help fight memory loss and improve the functionality of neurons. More studies show that an almond diet can reduce symptoms of Alzheimer's disease that is characterized by poor memory.

12. Wild fish

Fatty fish such as sardines, salmon, and herring contains high amounts of essential fatty acids. For instance, salmon has both high-quality protein as well as fatty acids, nutrients that are known to boost brain health and enhance the functionality of other cells. The fatty fish also has DHA and EPA, nutrients that control the synthesis of healthy brain cells, and can combat depression and bipolar disorder.

You need about 10 grams of this nutrient though taking at least 1g of EPA and DHA can work wonders if taken daily. Wild fish varieties also contain tryptophan, which is used to make serotonin. For people who don't like high omega 3 foods like mackerel, sardines or the salmon, you can take supplements which work in a similar manner wild fish.

13. Flaxseeds/ Flax oil

Both flaxseed and its oil can help boost the serotonin level due to the high concentration of both omega 3 fatty acids and that of tryptophan. Around 60 percent of your brain is made from structural fats such as omega 3 fatty acids; which has the highest proportion of the brain nerve cells. Research has shown that consuming about 1-2 tablespoons of flaxseed oil or 1-4 tablespoons of flaxseeds can help boost the mood, memory and other psychological problems. To boost memory and learning process, try combining processed flax oil into cottage cheese in order to make it soluble. Taking a soluble flaxseed combination helps improve its absorption and effectiveness of omega 3 fatty acids in the cells.

14. Oatmeal

Oatmeal has nutrients like potassium, zinc, vitamin B complex, and vitamin E, which have direct influence on your learning skills, brain longevity, and memory. This food also boasts a lot of soluble fiber that help regulate cholesterol level in the blood, and reduce the low-density lipoprotein. This bad cholesterol can accumulate in the blood vessels and disrupt flow of oxygen to the brain, leading to brain damage. On the other hand, oatmeal promotes satiety and reduces craving especially for people with blood sugar problems or those intending to shed off few pounds.

15. Free Range Turkey

Protein foods like turkey contain tryptophan, an amino acid that helps in synthesis of serotonin, a neurotransmitter. Eating free-range turkey can help maintain a healthy mental outlook through a correct balance of serotonin levels in the brain. After eating diet high in tryptophan, together with carbohydrates, all amino acids save for the tryptophan is cleared from the blood. The tryptophan is left to freely cross your brain barrier to constitute the serotonin neurotransmitter.

People who regularly report eating free-range turkey report feeling very relaxed and energetic due to improved functionality of serotonin. The meat is also high in essential fats, which are available in a well-balanced ratio. Eating a turkey alongside cranberry sauce sandwich with whole grain bread can boost learning process and brain function to optimum functionality.

16. Sweet Potatoes

Compared to regular white potatoes, sweet potatoes are more recommendable to due to less sugar content. Sweet potato has antioxidants that help fight inflammation, which can slow down the brain functions especially in people who suffer Alzheimer's disease. These potatoes also contain carotenoids, chemicals, which has ability to inhibit damage caused by free radicals. These chemicals also help in synthesis of new neurons and their connection to improve communication within the body.

On the other hand, baked white potato with its skin and no-added salt has health benefits that you need to boost memory and learning process. For example, 100 grams of baked potatoes offers about 16 percent of RDA for vitamin B6 and C, an 11 percent RDA for manganese and a 15 percent RDA for potassium. These minerals are known to enhance synthesis of brain chemicals among them GABA, melatonin and serotonin.

17. Turmeric

Turmeric root can help cure various brain defects due to presence of curcumin, a chemical compound that has anti-inflammatory properties. The spice also has antioxidant abilities and can improve immunity which boosting the amount of oxygen that reaches the brain. In so doing turmeric helps keep you alert and able to easily process information.

18. Tomatoes

The veggie is known to offer protection from free radicals that cause Alzheimer's disease and dementia. Tomato has high amount of lycopene, which help soak up and destroy free radicals before they cause serious damage to brain cells. Lycopene is responsible for the bright red color of tomatoes thus, you should rich for the ripe varieties. Research shows that cooked tomatoes have a higher content of the chemical and thus it's advisable to eat cooked tomatoes.

19. Brown rice

The best ways to supply enough energy for the brain functions is through consumption of whole grains. Eating whole but unprocessed grains offer glucose to the brain, which acts as fuel. Brown rice is rich in riboflavin, which is used to generate energy for the brain cells. You'll also benefit from other B vitamins among them niacin and thiamin which similarly plays a brain enhancement role. Try other whole grains like wheat bran; brown pasta; rolled oats and whole wheat bread to remain mentally focused the entire day.

20. Collard greens

These are rich in vitamin K, which can relieve symptoms of Alzheimer's disease. Collard greens work by inhibiting neuron damage in the brain. The veggie also has pyridoxine, pantothenic acid, riboflavin, and niacin, B vitamins, which boost brain power. The sprouts also contain various minerals that work in a similar manner such as iron, selenium, zinc, magnesium, and copper.

21. Cheese and yoghurt

Whether you consume swish, cheddar or ricotta cheese, you're to benefit from high quality proteins and other nutrients. Research shows that taking milk products like yoghurt, cheese, or unprocessed milk can boost the mental ability compared to other consuming no dairy at-all. However, it isn't well understood how cheese products can boost brain function or combat mental fatigue. On the other hand, the probiotics found in yoghurt can boost cognitive responses especially in brain parts involved in processing of sensation and emotion.

22. Soybeans

Legumes contain folate, a form of B vitamin, which helps lower the effect of amino acids that impairs brain functions. Legumes among them pinto beans, garbanzo beans, black beans, and lentils possess properties that boost brain power and memory. All legumes are nutritious but soybeans are recommendable legumes to start with.

In a research study, a Japanese firm found out that the protein in soybeans is beneficial for the brain. Participants who ate soybean peptide powder that was mixed with water were found to have higher levels of brain chemicals in their cerebral blood. Peptide or proteins found in soybeans can therefore boost the level of adrenaline and other neurotransmitters. Add more legumes to your dishes, soups, salads, and fries to ensure you get enough folate.

23. Brussels sprouts

These sprouts can offer the required vitamin K to boost brain power. Brussels sprouts also offer omega 3 fatty acids, vitamin C and tryptophan, which all help strengthen DNA cells and encourage optimal brain function.

24. Pumpkin seeds

These seeds are known for the presence of glutamate, a chemical compound that helps manufacture GABA. This is an anti-stress hormone that helps inhibit disruption in brain functions. Snack on a few of the seeds to get ample supply of B vitamins, which helps boost brain functionality.

25. Tart/ Sour Cherries

These are rich in melatonin, a hormone that promotes functionality of adrenal glands, boosts restful sleep and synthesis of serotonin. Obtaining a peaceful sleep can also help boost levels of serotonin neurotransmitter, thus melatonin works both ways to enhance mental function. Try eating around 20 red tart cherries or drink a glass of sour cherry juice before sleep, alongside ricotta or cottage cheese on rye bread. These foods boost serotonin levels during sleep and make you wake up refreshed and mentally fit.

26. Blackcurrant

This fruit has anthocyanins, which can boost alertness and concentration. The active ingredients are also able to fight negative symptoms of stress and fatigue to ensure a balanced cognitive response. A research study reveals that people who eat black currants regularly were generally less exhausted even after performing mentally draining tests that lasted for a few hours. The dark berries are also rich in vitamin C, in high concentration that is 5 times that of oranges! The vitamin can help inhibit burnout of brain cells and boost mental agility.

27. Bone Broth

Broth has vital benefits for your gut bacteria, which in turn promote a healthy brain. It has ample amounts of like proline and glycine amino acids, which has shown to boost memory, and enhance immune response. Bone broth also helps fight food allergies, leaky gut and can boost your joint health; while presence of collagen helps heal intestinal inflammation.

28. Grapes

The fruit is known to cure both the heart and the brain. Based on scientific studies, the polyphenols in grapes were found to increase memory and learning skills. These chemicals have shown to greatly boost the communication between brain cells. For instance, red grapes are delicious and favored ingredients in red wines due to the high quantity of resveratrol. This chemical has shown to heal disorders that affect the circulatory system, and can inhibit conditions Alzheimer's disease and dementia. If you don't take wine, munching a few red grapes can offer you similar benefits.

29. Whey Protein

This super food has shown to boost immune system and increase the levels of serotonin neurotransmitter. A recent study showed that eating a diet rich in whey protein could boost the plasma TrpLNAA, a benchmark that is used to measure serotonin function. Increase in the plasma TrpLNAA, is linked to better functioning of serotonin, and researchers confirmed that whey protein had potential to boost its production. Whey protein was found to boost the release of serotonin and tryptophan levels and thus lead to better mood and increased mental activity.

30. Pomegranates

Research studies show that pregnant women who take the pomegranate fruit are likely to give birth to infants with healthier brains; and that are not starved from oxygen. A related study reveals that the polyphenols found in the fruit can reduce the buildup of beta-amyloid, a substance that can cause the Alzheimer's disease.

Apart from the foods that help boost memory and accelerate the rate of learning or grasping things, these herbs are also recommended:

Herbs that boost memory and learning

1. Chamomile

Chamomile oil contains a-bisabolol chemical, which possesses anti-inflammatory and antispasmodic properties. Problems such as stress and inflammation slow down the brain and delay learning process. The herb is effective in dealing with stress as well as calming the nerves especially in dosages of one to three 6-ounce mugs of tea; equivalent to 400 to 1600 mg daily. Try incorporating the herb in tea or another beverage to reduce tension and maintain your brain health.

2. Cinnamon

Cinnamon contains proanthocyanidins and cinnamaldehyde compounds, which have potential to prevent buildup of harmful proteins. For instance, there can be buildup of tau proteins that are known to inhibit the brain functionality. These tau proteins slow down and finally kill brain cells, and lead to Alzheimer's disease. You can add a dash of cinnamon to your cake, oatmeal or bread to improve brain function and general health.

3. Rosemary

The herb contains carnosic acid, which research shows can prevent the brain from undergoing neurodegeneration. Rosemary helps to fight free radicals that cause damage to the brain thereby immature death of brain neurons. On the other hand, the herb can help fight stroke, Alzheimer's disease and promote healthy aging of the brain. You can also get other benefits like improved eyesight due to the anti-inflammatory and antioxidant properties of rosemary.

4. Holy Basil

Holy basil leaf extract contains a synergistic effect with silymarin, the active ingredient that is made of various flavonoids. Research has shown that taking holy basil is effective for reducing brain failure as the herb hinders build-up of cortisol hormone. The herb can also improve cerebral circulation and memory, while at the same time relieving cloudy thinking and general mental fog. Holy basil can also treat attention deficit disorder, attention deficit hyperactivity disorder and other forms of depression.

5. Ginseng

Having a good mental health contributes to the anti-aging effect, and ginseng has an ability to reduce degeneration of the blood stream, as well as improving learning process. Ginseng root contains panaxosides or ginsenosides, active ingredients that are responsible for the medicinal properties. This herb has been found to improve the memory and mental performance, while stimulating the immune system and the lowering the blood cholesterol.

Ginseng is suitable for you in fighting fatigue, effects of stress, cholesterol levels and preventing infections. The herb is also effective in treating problems such as anxiety, improving resistance to stress and depression. These mood disorders are known to affect your brain functionality and slow down learning and cognitive response.

6. Sage

This herb has excellent medicinal properties on the brain in addition to its unique taste when added to dishes. Research shows that people who consume about 50 micro liters of sage oil often perform better on cognitive tests than those who don't. The active ingredients in sage work by inhibiting breakdown of memory, and in the process boost the function of acetylcholine, a neurotransmitter.

7. Bacopa

This herb originates from India and has been confirmed effective in improving memory, learning and cognition response. The herb contains triterpene glycosides; substances, which enhance the efficiency in transmission of nerve impulses. The herb also contains antioxidant properties, which offer protection against brain damage. Taking a bacopa liquid herbal extract will provide you with benefits such as improved cognitive function, focus, and emotional well being.

Conclusion

Learning is as volatile a thing as camphor. You cannot put leash on your ability to learn just to control it according to your whims. However, what we learnt in this book tells us a different tale. We learnt that despite how fickle our minds are, we could always tame it to make it our slave.

The suggestions, tips, strategies and methods so written in this book are proven techniques, tried and tested by many like you. Learning issues are common, more so among students. Many complain of an inability to learn well and hence deteriorating academic results. The third chapter of this book illustrated and explained how memory, as an important part of learning, can be not just sharpened but turned into a clever servant. The fourth chapter touches a topic that is usually ignored when it comes to offering help with a bad memory.

Imagination is the solutions to a lot of things and memory problem is one of them. Remember, only ten percent of your brain's memory is used by you. The rest ninety percent is just dormant memory lying around. If you manage to upgrade even five percent of the available ten, you have successfully mastered your memory. The other remaining chapters offered different methods of accelerating your learning potential, including lifestyle and reading – two often-neglected aspects of learning.

Thank you for purchasing the book. I hope you enjoyed reading it, and that it was both informative and fun.

Learning

Bonus

Thanks for making it this far in your education. If you want the real multiplier effect and to take your skills and effectiveness to the next level, I recommend the easy-to-follow quick tips below.

CLICK HERE: Top 10 Productivity Tips & Hacks GUARANTEED to Unlock Massive Amounts of Time, Crush Decision Fatigue, and Skyrocket Your Efficiency and Effectiveness

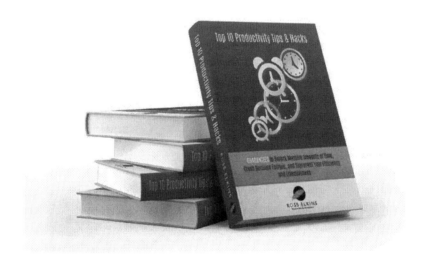

Link: https://funnelb.leadpages.co/smarter-not-harder-business/

Made in the USA
Lexington, KY
02 July 2019